THE SHIFTING SOURCES
OF POWER AND INFLUENCE

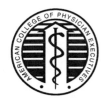

American College of Physician Executives
Two Urban Centre, Suite 200
4890 West Kennedy Blvd.
Tampa, Florida 33609-2575
813/287-2000

ISBN: 0-924674-12-1

Library of Congress Catalog Card Number: 92-74648

Printed in the United States of America by Rinaldi Printing Co., Tampa, Florida.

Competition and conflict, power and influence. Organizations are dominated by the tensions among these forces. And organizations are the medium by which cultures, and individuals, attend to their needs, particularly in our modern, industrialized, information-driven society.

In this new book from the American College of Physician Executives, Charles Dwyer, PhD, of the University of Pennsylvania, makes a strong case for the view that organizations are no more than collections of individuals. It is the behaviors and values of the individuals who belong to the organization that drive the organization and its course. The organization itself has no persona. It does not live.

A significant aspect of personal success in organizations is the ability to identify and control seats of power and influence. To do so, he says, you first have to understand both your values and the values of those around you. When all those values are clear in your mind, and only then, you can move to the more rewarding task of appealing to the values of others in order to influence them to change their behaviors in a way that satisfies your values.

The physician executive's ability to influence people will be this professional's greatest attribute in the move into more and more powerful positions within medical management. But the dynamics of influence are not nearly as simple as they sound. In this monograph, Dr. Dwyer lays out in great detail just how influence can be gained, and used, in the pursuit of organizational power.

Roger Schenke
Executive Vice President
American College of Physician Executives
Tampa, Florida
October 31, 1992

Charles Dwyer, PhD, has been on the faculty of the University of Pennsylvania since 1966. He has held positions as Chairman of the Board of the Wharton Center for Applied Research, Director of Wharton's Management and Behavioral Science Center, and Faculty Coordinator for Wharton's Effective Executive Development Programs. At present, he chairs the Educational Leadership Division of the Graduate School of Education. He has more than 30 years of experience in corporate and organizational consulting and in executive education, including the design of Wharton's well-known Effective Executive Workshop. His client list includes IBM, Dupont, Xerox, AT&T, General Electric, the New York Stock Exchange, Polaroid, Texaco, General Mills, Pepsi-Cola, Caterpillar, Pitney Bowes, the Buick Division of General Motors, RJR/Nabisco, Mercedes Benz, Merck Sharpe & Dohme, Intel, Bates Advertising, the Justice Department, the General Services Administration, and the Federal Reserve System.

In addition, Professor Dwyer founded and is Chairman of the Board of the Swarthmore Academy, a private, not-for-profit, college preparatory school in Swarthmore, Pa. The Academy focuses on rigorous and challenging learning; substantive student experiences both as entrepreneurs and as interns in organizations; the use of computers in learning; and the creation, testing, and dissemination of concepts designed to facilitate the development of self-reliant, successful, and contributing adults.

Dr. Dwyer's research and teaching cover a wide variety of topics, including human influence, motivation, dealing with difficult people, productivity improvement, quality of work life, self-management, conflict resolution, problem resolution, leadership, organizational design, organizational change, entre/intrapreneurship, selling, risk taking, creativity, team building, group processes, personal development, and organizational ethics.

Professor Dwyer received his bachelor's degree in economics from St. Joseph's University and his master's degree in organizational behavior and industrial relations and his doctorate in philosophy and education from Cornell University. He is a charter member of the faculty of the American College of Physician Executives. This monograph is based in part on his presentations at the College Physician in Management Seminar ll on the subject of power and influence in organizations.

CONTENTS

CHAPTER ONE

THE SHIFT IN
VALUE SYSTEMS

Our lives are centered on influence and influencing. Nearly everything we do all day long—in our work, with our families, in our recreation, in all of our varied environments—is, in one way or another, an attempt to influence the behavior of the people around us—the behavior of patients, patients' families, staff, physicians, volunteers, administrators, legislators, third-party payers, pharmacists. For physicians, this is a considerable change. In the "good old days," physicians received pretty much whatever they wanted. The world responded to them in terms of their profession and their positions. In the growth years after the end of World War II, there were more and more resources and unprecedented economic growth. We wanted more health care, more physicians, more hospitals. Physicians received respect, deference, and the budgets they wanted. They had little need for influence. It was theirs for the taking.

As the saying goes, "the times they are a changing." Since the end of World War II, great changes have been occurring in every element of society—families, marriages, interpersonal relationships generally, neighborhoods, schools, hospitals, government entities, private industries, and businesses. The same changes that are apparent at the global level in international affairs are also apparent in individual lives. The turmoil in health care is simply a manifestation of what is happening everywhere.

Increasingly, what is involved in understanding the changes and their consequences, and in what we can do about them, is human influence. It is necessary to secure cooperation and collaboration instead of anger and hostility, conflict and dysfunctional competition. I am certainly not against all conflict, nor am I against all competition. There is a great deal of conflict that is highly productive, desirable, even essential. There is also a great deal of it that isn't particularly productive. Most organizations suffer from too little of the right kind of conflict and competition and too much of the wrong kind.

The same may be said for interpersonal and international relationships. Wherever there are issues of conflict versus cooperation, the tool for resolution is human influence. The goal should be to improve your capability to engage in behaviors that will be effective in influencing the behavior of other people—to know what do to and how to do it in the various organizations within which you operate—so that you can get the desired patterns of behavior from the people you wish to influence.

There is a great deal of misinformation in the world about conflict and cooperation. I think there is generally a great deal of unnecessary mystification as to what human behavior and human influence are all about. Much of the responsibility for this state of affairs may be laid at the doorstep of academia. Academics live, move, and breath on complications. One of the things I learned many years ago in academia is that the more we jargonize, confuse, and obfuscate in our communication, the longer our academic careers are likely to be. The more un-understandable we are, the more likely we are to be published. It is necessary to cut through much of that fog and find some fundamental notions of what human behavior and human influence, as well as conflict and cooperation, are all about. It is also essential to explain these terms so as to give a sense of what seems irrational or unexplainable in human behavior.

The patterns of behavior that I engage in at the University of Pennsylvania now to maintain my effectiveness are quite different from what they were 27 years ago when I started. The same is true everywhere. For example, we now must work at what we used to get by default. We now have to take time, energy, and personal resources and devote them to activities that we don't necessarily find inherently satisfying. Such activities are required if we are to maintain and, indeed, add to our ability to get what we want out of our organizations. In understanding these changes, we begin where they began, shortly after the end of World War II. Again, this is just a frame, a way of understanding. But our frames, our ways of understanding, eventually determine the patterns of our behavior, and the patterns of our behavior determine our effectiveness.

Two things had to happen simultaneously for us to be facing the challenges that we face today:

• Value fragmentation or heterogeneity of values.

• Diffusion of power.

It has always been true that different peoples have had very different notions of right and wrong, good and bad, satisfying and unsatisfying, obligation and prohibition.

The Shift in Value Systems

World War II brought these differences to a head, because it brought peoples in contact with others who had exceedingly different views of these fundamental notions. Generally increased levels of education, of affluence, and of travel have exacerbated this trend. The technology of communication, particularly television, multiplies the intensity of it by bringing conflicting value systems forcefully to our attention every day.

When I was born in 1937, my world was extraordinarily homogeneous in terms of value messages, of belief messages. Everybody told me just about the same thing concerning what was right, what was wrong, what was good, what was bad, who I was, where I fit in. As a consequence, I was able to develop a series of quite confident beliefs about right, wrong, good, bad, etc. After World War II, the game plan changed. I really do wonder how someone born today, or even 15 or 20 years ago, can come to confident beliefs, because, almost from the moment of birth, they have been inundated with well-packaged, well-delivered messages in conflict. Messages attempting to fill up their belief space about what is right and wrong, good and bad, satisfying and unsatisfying, what happiness consists in, what expectations they are to have about the world, what their responsibilities are.

How do you decide what to believe in a world where you are bombarded with contrasting and conflicting messages about fundamental beliefs? If you are a 16-year-old, you may decide to simply throw up your hands in despair of ever coming to confident beliefs. How can a child understand what he or she ought to believe—about capital punishment, abortion, pro-life, pro-choice, war? Is there such a thing as a just war? Should we or should we not do "X" and, if so, under what conditions? All sorts of fundamental issues are now uncertain. And there is confusion in interpersonal issues. How am I to treat other people, what is honesty all about, what are my expectations, what are my obligations, what are other peoples obligations to me? We have more people more aware of the differences they have with others in their fundamental belief systems than we have ever had before, and there is no end in sight. Beliefs are becoming even more fragmented now that we have greatly multiplied channels of television from which to choose, plus videotapes, audiotapes, and myriad additional technologies for delivering messages to people.

Value heterogeneity in and of itself doesn't necessarily create the seeds of dysfunctional conflict. It is only a piece. Something else has to happen simultaneously—the diffusion of power. Power is more diffused than it has ever been before. More people have more power than they have ever had before in the history of humankind. I am not saying that this is a monolithic trend. There are always people pushing in the opposite direction, people trying to hold onto centralized power, but on the whole, what we see in the world is the diffusion of power.

What do I mean by diffusion of power? As an example, in our society, who has more power as a group than they did 25 years ago, both as individuals and as individuals within groups. Elderly, minorities, consumers, women, the handicapped, children, young people. A participant in one of my seminars came up to me at a break and told me a story about the power of children. He was away on a business trip and called his wife the night he reached his destination. She was quite upset. She and their 12-year-old son had had another argument, apparently a recurring event. The son was rushing out of the house, and the wife said he had to clean his room first. The son had had all day to accomplish this task and hadn't done it. His response was that he had to leave to play ball. He had to get to the field by 4 o'clock. She was firm, and the argument intensified. He was giving her a lot of lip, and she lost her temper and slapped him across the face.

Here we come to the diffusion of power. The participant told his wife he understood why she was upset, but she told him that he didn't understand. She said that their son went to his room after the slap, she thought to clean the room. Not so. He went to his room and called the child abuse hot line. Twenty minutes later, two people from the child abuse agency were at the door interviewing the son about child abuse. They promised to come back every two weeks for the next six months to check on abuse. Could you imagine, when you were 12 years old, if you even had a phone in your room, "blowing the whistle" on your parents over such an incident? That son has social service agencies available to him at 12 years of age. He has a way to influence the behavior of his parents.

Power is more diffused in our society and around the world. Before the Persian Gulf War, Iraq had the fourth largest military establishment in the world. China, the Soviet Union, the United States, and then Iraq. That is power. There have been terrorists for thousands of years, certainly hundreds of years, but they weren't as much of a problem as they are today. Terrorists can move easily around the world using weapons of great destructive force. Because of modern communication systems, terrorists high-jack a plane and, within 30 minutes, anybody within a hundred yards of a television or radio knows who they are and what they want. That's power.

In the United States' legal system, the contingency fee has done more to democratize the law and diffuse power than anything I can think of in the history of the law. If people don't have access to the law, it is useless to them. The

The Shift in Value Systems

contingency fee gave people access to the law. It gave them the ability to influence decisions, behavior, and the allocation of societal resources. That's power.

Who has gained power in the health care system of the United States? Patients, nurses, pharmacists, legislators, courts, third-party payers, and even software designers. This is part of what is complicating your life.

One more dimension must be added to this. If, on the one hand, we see value fragmentation and heterogeneity—more and more people with differing views of what is right and wrong, good and bad, satisfying and unsatisfying—and on the other hand, diffusion of power—people having the capability of acting on their differing beliefs and values and, added to this we have a fixed set of resources called Earth, what might you expect as a consequence? Conflict. Interpersonal, intergroup, interregional, international conflict.

These days you can assemble a support group for your values virtually at the drop of a headline. It doesn't seem to matter how absurd the cause is. A group of people will band together to bring their collective power to bear on the issue and ask for resources. Contributing to the potential for conflict in all this is the fact that too few in this society seem to have been brought up to think about trade-offs. If we do this, what is it we are not going to do? If we are going to put more research dollars into AIDS, what should we take it away from? What other diseases shouldn't we look at? Should we take money away from research on cancer, heart disease, Alzheimer's? There is no concern for trade-offs or compromises. There is a fixed set of resources, and each group focuses solely on enlarging or at least maintaining what it sees as its share.

The elderly are a good example of such an interest group. As the graying of the population continues and the elderly gain more and more power (e.g., an ability to influence Congress), who are they going to be taking resources away from? It isn't said baldly, but the answer is, among others, young people. Why? Because young people don't have the leverage that older people have in terms of control of resources, of voting patterns, of overall effective influence behaviors of various kinds.

Value heterogeneity and power diffusion are not likely to be altered in the near term. They will have to be dealt with. To be effective, managers, and physician executives, will have to use influence to achieve the patterns of behavior that are more consonant with their own values. In the following chapters, I will outline a model that can lead to more effective management of dissonant values in a world of diffused power and intense competition for limited resources.

5

CHAPTER TWO

A Little
Background Music

It is not easy to process the immense quantity of information coming at us and then choose effective behaviors. We have to develop conceptual frameworks for that information that will help us process it, make sense of it, in advance of action. We likewise need greater sensitivity to the assumptions we make. We each have such frameworks and assumptions in our heads, but they tend to be subconscious, fuzzy, or tacit. Nonetheless, no matter how submerged these frameworks may be, they eventually control our behavior, which, in turn, determines our effectiveness. A story will illustrate my point.

Two fellows were camping overnight beside a mountain stream for the first time. They came in late at night, went to sleep, and got up at the crack of dawn. Cold as the water was, they waded in barefooted and started fishing for salmon, having a good time. Suddenly, they hear a great roar behind them and turn to face a grizzly bear. They drop their fishing gear, head for the near bank, instinctively grab their socks and sneakers, and start running barefoot up the other side. Despite the fact that they are in great physical shape, the gap between them and the bear slowly but surely diminishes. Suddenly, one of them stops and calmly starts to put on his socks and sneakers. His friend stops and, in a panic, asks him what he's doing. The friend points out that the bear is almost upon them and suggests that putting on socks and sneakers isn't going to help him outrun the bear. The stopped runner replies that he has just realized he doesn't have to outrun the bear, only his friend. That is called "reframing the problem."

It is also an illustration of how we process data and of how our models direct our behavior and thus determine our effectiveness. If we don't begin to think in terms of a world of heterogeneous values, diffused power, and fixed resources, we will more and more expend our energies fighting fruitless rear guard actions. All those other actors on the health care scene will keep scratching away at our turf and increase

7

their power relative to us. As they chip away, our frustration will grow and our effectiveness will decline.

What are the alternatives? There are some who would propose to forcefully homogenize values. They would tell everybody their "truth." They are right and others are wrong. They would also centralize power—in them. Homogenization of values requires indoctrination, brainwashing, and persuasion and violates two fundamental American values—pluralism and self-determination. You have to give those up if you are going to homogenize values and bring everybody to a single truth. As for centralization of power, Lord Acton's observation that power tends to corrupt and absolute power tends to corrupt absolutely is apt.

As it turns out, there are some alternatives that do not involve homogenization and centralization. They are complicated, sophisticated, and costly, but they are extraordinarily effective. They are based on increasing our ability to influence human behavior in a world of increased complexity. The "bad news" about power and influence is that there is no magic in getting people to do what you want them to do, and there are some personal risks in doing so. The good news is that changing people's behavior doesn't require any esoteric knowledge or special skill, only the willingness to do what is necessary.

We have a thirst for magical, no-cost, no-risk, guaranteed ways of influencing human behavior. Anyone who has been victimized by an overzealous application of management by objectives, zero-base budgeting, matrix management, quality control circles, autonomous work groups, job rotation, job enlargement, job enrichment, industrial democracy, participative management, or strategic planning knows about the search for magical management answers. Total quality management (or continuous quality improvement) is the latest potion to be touted in health care. I'm not opposed to these ideas. In fact, I use some of them in my consulting work. The difficulty is that they are often taught, and, I fear, even more often endorsed and embraced, as the ultimate way of changing behavior. "Get the right incentive system! Get the proper organizational structure!" and everything will finally be taken care of in terms of human influence. It does not work that way.

The truth. There is no simple, magical, structural, answer to the issues of human influence. It isn't likely that tomorrow IBM or The Wharton School or the Defense Department is going to come up with a definitive answer on how to get people to do what you want them to do. I'm reminded of the seminars whose organizers assure the public that attendees are going to make millions with the advice that will be offered. Why aren't those offering the advice out in the world following their own advice instead of creating competitors for themselves? Must be altruism!

Risk is the other part of the bad news. The number one barrier to quantum leaps in getting cooperation, collaboration, and synergy from the people around you is your reluctance to do what works. There are quite specific costs and risks implicit in the techniques that work. And we will examine them in detail.

We learn some very powerful behaviors for influencing others when we are two and three years old. We have to. We are dependent on other people to take care of what is important to us, so we have to find ways of getting parents, brothers and sisters, and other people in our worlds to do what we want them to do. And yet we eliminate or significantly reduce the effectiveness of those behaviors as we grow older. They are socially acceptable and extraordinarily powerful, and yet we rely less and less on them. Why? Because we begin to experience the costs and risks associated with them, particularly ego costs and risks. Indeed, we may be at the peak of our interpersonal power at age three, and it is likely that we all go down hill from then on.

As noted above, the good news is much shorter than the bad news, as it almost always is. Getting others to do what you want doesn't require special skill. You already have most of the knowledge that you need to take that quantum leap in interpersonal effectiveness. You can, almost immediately, be more effective with your spouse, your children, and your colleagues. I will describe some skills and their application throughout this book. Whether or not you will use them and be more effective is a decision you have to make. I once stopped a commercial airliner in motion at the Philadelphia airport to let me on. I did not throw my body in front of the plane. I didn't threaten, deceive, or bribe anyone. I used tried and true methods of influencing human behavior. What's more, I achieved my purposes in a socially acceptable, honest, and moral way. I'll relate that incident a little later as an illustration of an application of the concepts of this book.

While influence techniques are simple and powerful, they're not easy. They're not cost-free, risk-free, or guaranteed. Their use may be particularly difficult for those who have been in health care for a long time and remember when it was easy and probably relatively low cost and low risk to get people to do what you want. Those days are gone, and they are not likely to return.

There is another point that needs to be explored before we get to the actual techniques for influencing behavior. I said earlier that how we think about things, how we frame them, determines our patterns of behavior, and our patterns of behavior determine our effectiveness. That fact is universal. Human influence techniques operate in all environments and within all interpersonal relationships. They cover marketing, advertising, sales, merchandising, politics, religion, parenting, spousing, negotiation, conflict avoidance, and conflict resolution. They are useful in dealing with a waiter or waitress in a restaurant, a clerk in a store, a teller at the bank, a flight attendant on an airliner, a next-door neighbor, or a mechanic who works on your car. Any single individual or group of individuals whom you are trying to influence is covered by these techniques. The principles of human influence are generic. Each instance in which they are applied ultimately involves some individual attempting to use his or her behavior to influence the behavior of one or more other individuals.

I am not describing behaviorist theory here. I am stressing values—internal states, perceptions, human information processes. When I am trying to influence an individual or a group, one of the things I do is focus on what behavior or performance I want from that individual or group. Something observable, measurable, and quantifiable. We have not been taught to think that way. We have been taught to express our desires concerning other people in vague, general terms. Try to remember how, in the recent past, you thought about what you wanted from someone else. How did you verbalize your wishes? Think of situations that involved people whom you would like to influence and get cooperation from, people with whom you have dysfunctional, counterproductive conflict. Think of how you talked to yourself about what you want from those people. What words did you use to express what you wanted from your boss, your peers, your subordinates, or your children? Respect? Cooperation? Support? More creativity? More production? Higher Quality? Loyalty, commitment, synergy? These are not very effective ways to talk or think if influence is the goal. But that is what we have been taught. "I want more autonomy from my boss, I want more cooperation from my colleagues, I want more support from my subordinates."

What is the problem with these ways of thinking and speaking? They are too vague, too general. They are not observable, measurable, or quantifiable. When you say you want more respect or more loyalty or more support or more cooperation, what is the evidence that the person or group is not already what you want them to be, doing what will serve your values? What is the evidence that you are not getting the loyalty, commitment, autonomy, and cooperation that you want? The people with whom we deal send out a few data fragments of behavior, these data points hit our sensors, they roll around in our central processing units, and then we reach grandiose conclusions. We attribute all kinds of motivations and generalized behavior to them on the basis of a few data fragments. When you try to influence these people, what is your evidence of success or failure? A few data fragments of behavior. We start and end with behavior, and in between we have been taught to get our heads all fuzzied up with attitudes, dispositions, personality characteristics, vague descriptors of relationships, and assumed motivations of others.

How might all this affect our behavior toward others in our attempts to influence them? An everyday event will illustrate the point. Suppose that I am very dissatisfied with the way the newspaper boy is delivering my paper. I stop him on a Saturday morning and say, "In the future I want my paper timely, readable, and conveniently placed. Is that clear?" What does the kid say: "No, stupid." Of course not. He says, "Yes, sir. That's clear." Of course, he continues his old pattern of behavior, because he thought that he was already meeting those criteria. He doesn't know what I mean by "timely," "readable," and "conveniently placed." If I say I want the paper delivered no later than six a.m., neatly folded in order, dry, neither smeared nor torn, and placed between my storm door and regular door, I have at least some chance of getting that outcome.

We frequently do not act with this sharpness of focus toward others, and then we wonder why we have been ineffective. You don't like the way the receptionist answers the phone. "She should," you say "be more sympathetic, more helpful, and more supportive of our patients." That doesn't mean anything to the receptionist. You may know what that means to you, but you probably haven't taken the time to determine what the data fragments of the receptionist's behavior are that lead you to want her to change and what specific alterations you want in the receptionist's behavior. That takes work and discipline that we don't want to invest. But if you don't make the investment, you are not creating a target worthy of your efforts. Until you discipline yourself to think in terms of specific, concrete behaviors and measurable performances, you are not likely to increase your effectiveness in dealing with those around you.

There is one other point that deserves attention before I get to the nitty-gritty of influence. What is it that I have available to me to influence any of the 5.3 billion people on earth? What do I have available to me to influence world leaders or my dean or my colleagues or my family? The only resource that I know of to influence anybody else is my behavior. Directly or indirectly, all I have to influence the behavior of anyone else on the face of the earth are the data fragments of my own behavior. What I say, how I say it, the words that I use, the rhythm, the tone, the timing, the gesture, the mode of communication, these are my tools. Do I go one-on-one? Do I talk to you on the phone, do I send you a memo, do I try to influence you through a group meeting, do I try to influence you through someone else? If you want to increase your ability to get cooperation out of people, you have to look much more self-consciously, much more critically at your own behavior. There is no way to increase your effectiveness without changing the patterns of your behavior. We need to determine how the patterns of our own behavior must be altered if we wish to increase our ability to get what we want from the people around us.

You may wonder, with all of the time, energy, and brilliance that has gone into the study of human behavior, particularly over the past 50 years, why we aren't better at it. Why do we still have dysfunctional conflicts? If we are so smart about human behavior, why haven't we been doing the things described here? There continues to be a great deal of talk about worker productivity in the United States. About how worried we are and how the Japanese and the Germans and maybe the Koreans are overtaking us in terms of productivity. The means to increase worker productivity in this country have been known and empirically documented for more than 30 years. If knowing how to get workers to do more of what you want them to do is not difficult, why aren't we doing it? It is no big mystery at all. It's because the means of accomplishing the increase threaten the values of the people who have to implement them. Most people who say that they want more power to influence refuse to do what works; if they did what we already know is effective, productivity would quickly and dramatically increase.

My most effective intervention in an organization to date helped produce a 68 percent increase in productivity in 8 months. This was a plant in an 11-plant company, and it was sixth in productivity at the beginning of the intervention Within 8 months, it was first, and it still is 7 years later. Quality went up, scrap went down, absenteeism went down, turnover went down, grievances went down, productivity went through the roof. Why? Because the plant manager was willing to do what was necessary. The vice president of human resources, who hired me to do this work, was astonished at the improvement. He took me to the president of the company, a closely held, family-owned firm. The vice president of human resources explained the results and asked where I should be sent next. The president and owner of the company said the one plant was enough. Why? Because my way of increasing productivity threatened some of his fundamental values, and he wasn't about to have me go to his other plants challenging his cherished beliefs no matter how great the potential productivity increases might be.

In the next chapter, I will discuss concepts of organization—how our concepts, beliefs, current frames and assumptions demonstrate themselves in our behaviors. Much of what we take for granted about how organizations operate and behave is, I think, obviously wrong. We have been given faulty frameworks. I will show how erroneous assumptions about the organization handicap us in efforts to change behaviors.

CHAPTER THREE

LIES, DAMNED LIES, AND ORGANIZATIONS

IBM, AT&T, General Motors, Unilever, the Catholic Church, the United Nations, a garden club, a bridge club, a friendship. What is it that these seemingly disparate entities could possibly have in common that would make it legitimate to call each of them an organization? In other words, what are the essential characteristics of an organization? Is it a group of people with a common interest? Is it a structure with defined relationships, assignments of authority and responsibility, rules, regulations, policies, practices, forms, and formats? Is it a matter of shared values, goals, mission, structure, a history, a culture. Is it a question of resources, people, materials, supplies, equipment, facilities? Do organizations require leaders? You probably believe that these are the elements, the pieces of the organization. Then, how do they fit together? What are the relationships among these elements? What is the dominant element that determines which are the appropriate resources and how resources are to be used in the organization and how the various elements are to be structured into various relationships?

The traditional notion of organizations suggests that each is driven by some desired outcome, the objective or goal, the purpose of the organization. That concept has been magnified in recent years by use of the notion of organizational mission, which, while it is relatively new, is pervasive. It connotes a religious association— you have been chartered by God and you are on some sort of a holy quest. The organizational lexicon has even sprouted a newer term—vision. Presumably, you don't need a mission if you have vision, because now you are dealing direct. I have speculated as to what word in the organizational jargon would surpass vision in popularity. The only thing that I think could possibly qualify would be revelation. One day the CEO will walk in and say, "God gave me the budget." He or she will then open a brief case, take out two tablets, and explain the new budget. We used to just have goals and objectives, but we have gone well beyond that now.

So the organizational model goes something like this. The organization has a mission, a vision, objectives, goals, philosophies, ideals, ideologies, and values that serve as the organizational culture. It is the culture that tells the organization which resources to seek and use—people, knowledge, skills, facilities, supplies, materials. It is these desired outcomes and principles that tell us how to structure and organize the resources into various relationships and hierarchies so that the resources will interact to fulfill the mission of the organization. That has a geometric symmetry, a harmony, a seductive, esthetic quality to it. It is a somewhat simplified, but I don't think oversimplified, description. This is the organizational model most of us were brought up on. It is the model of organization you will find implicit, sometimes explicit, in everything you hear and read about organizations. It is the model of organization you will find implicit in any story in newspapers or news magazines. It is the organizational model that virtually all my colleagues in the field of management assume to be true.

The only difficulty with this model is that it's false, partial, and inadequate. It's myopic, counterproductive, and dysfunctional. It leads us astray in our search for behaviors that will help us influence others. I am not splitting hairs here. This is not some fine semantic distinction. Our models guide our behavior, and our behavior determines our effectiveness. We have been taught to behave in certain ways because of this model of organization, and such behavior, based on the model, is largely ineffective. Part of what is wrong with this model is that it imputes characteristics to the organization that it cannot have, characteristics that lead us to believe and act in certain ways toward others in the organization. This traditional model suggests that managers have to take the values of the individuals and the values of the organization and harmonize them. That is an impossibility. Those who have deviant values have to be brought aboard, they have to come around and buy into the values of the organization. The organizational model tends to be top down. Although my theorist colleagues continue to build both "top down" and "bottom up" and even horizontal models of organization, they persist in making the same flawed assumptions about the shared interests, shared values, and common purposes of the people in and around organizations.

The traditional organization model is upside down, inside out, and backwards. To put it as crisply as I can, organizations do not have, never have had, never will have, and indeed cannot have, in any meaningful sense, objectives, goals, purposes, missions, visions, ideals, ideologies, philosophies, or values. But we pretend that they do. The model pretends that organizations are living, moving, breathing, conscious entities. They are not purpose-seeking entities at all. They are none of the things that we say they are. We pretend that organizations are people. Indeed, in 1886, the Supreme Court of the United States declared that corporations are legal persons. That decision has never been overturned. Why? Because the people who owned those organizations wanted the protection of the Constitution of the United States to be extended to their fabrications and inventions. For the past 100 years, throughout the industrialized world, people have pretended that organizations are living, moving, breathing, conscious, entities—that organizations are people. It's the same fiction that causes people to say that organizations care deeply about their own survival. They don't (more properly IT doesn't). If any of the people in your organization ever tell you that the organization doesn't care about them, believe them. The organization doesn't care about anybody or anything. We not only have been seduced by this language, but also collude in its use because it's helpful to us in a limited and distorted way.

One of our favorite phrases is, "The organization is responsible." That means nobody is responsible. The headmaster of the academy I founded came to me a couple of years ago and said, with some righteousness in his voice, that the faculty had a right, was entitled to certain benefits that he listed for me. I responded that one of the things I discovered early on in my studies in ethics is that whenever anyone has a right, someone else has to have a corresponding obligation. An obligation to see to the protection and fulfillment of rights. When he agreed, I asked who had the responsibility for seeing to it that the rights of the teachers were met. He responded by saying "the Swarthmore Academy," so I told him to ask the Academy for the necessary funding. He paused and said that would be me, as Founder, Chairman of the Board, Chief Contributor, and Chief Fund Raiser. I agreed that it meant me, and then I rejected the notion that I had any such responsibility.

The problem with ascribing human characteristics to an organization is that it insulates people from the impact of their decisions. In the heyday of the Industrial Revolution, newspapers would report that Rockefeller was doing this, Carnegie was doing that, Mellon was doing some other thing. People were actually engaged in making decisions and having responsibilities for their outcomes. Some of the powerful people who were identified as making these decisions weren't too comfortable with this, so they hired a press agent who began issuing a new kind of press release on their behalf. Now the reports said the New York Central Railroad has decided, Standard Oil of New Jersey is about to, U.S. Steel is on its way to. All of a sudden, corporations, not people, were doing things. Again, this is not merely a semantic distinction. Let me offer a pragmatic implication. Do you think there might be any difference in prime-time television programming if the people responsible for the programming had to put their names on it. Instead of "CBS Presents," we would have had "William S. Paley Jr. proudly presents 'The Dukes of Hazard.'"

Of course, personification of organizations is a two-edged sword. It is much easier to take negative and hostile action toward a corporate person than it is toward an individual person. You don't invite organizations to your home for dinner. The organization's kids don't play with your kids. People can take incredibly negative action toward organizations and feel no guilt or concern. "I'm not hurting anybody; I'm just taking something away from big business." In the same vein, they see themselves as taking it away from the hospital or the insurance company, not from the staff, the nurses, or subsequent patients.

Organizations are created by human beings, but they are not human. And they arise in response to needs, but the needs are individual human needs, not community or societal needs. Organizations begin in people's heads. If you seriously question the assumption that organizations arise out of social needs, you will immediately see how phony the notion is. Many needs in the world go unanswered, and sometimes people create needs for products and services of a given organization. All organizations start with a single individual saying that the creation of some aggregation of resources (the organization) is the best way to take care of what is important to him or her. Organizations are always and everywhere nothing more than means, tools, and instrumentalities. They are never ends. They are not interested in their own survival. Sometimes there are people who are interested in the survival of an organization, sometimes not. And there are often people interested in the destruction, termination, elimination, or disintegration of an organization. Organizations are artifacts created by human beings. They are fabrications, conveniences, conventions, inventions—nothing more. They are temporary arrangements designed and run to take care of the values of the people who act in and around them—nothing more.

Where did the Ford Motor Company come from? Henry Ford. What was Henry up to? Making money. Why? Let's go beyond the instrumental value called money. What was Henry Ford ultimately after. Power, visibility, all sorts of things related to his ego. He wanted approval, acceptance, recognition, appreciation, gratitude, excitement, challenge, achievements, success, security, autonomy, satisfaction of curiosity. The purpose of money is precisely to give an individual a sense of security, of recognition and autonomy and fun and achievement and success. It is a means for the satisfaction of intrinsic human values. But, how did Ford get people to join him and create this organization? He needed investors, executives, managers, engineers. He needed suppliers of goods and services. He needed a distribution network and customers. The current mythology says he created a vision and other people shared it. "Joe, I'm Henry Ford and I have this dream. I'm going to supply low-cost, reliable transportation to the people of America, and I want you on my team. I do have to warn that you'll be working 80 hours a week. I can't pay you, and I'm certainly not going to share any equity in this organization, but we're talking a dream. What do you say?"

That is the Hollywood version of what organizations are all about. Shared goals, shared path, common interest, common values. Creation of an organizational culture, complete with values, etc., and getting people to buy into it. What is more, this is the language that people in organizations use publicly to define the organization. It is the stuff of mission statements and organizational cultures. People (not organizations) are spending hundred of thousands of dollars, sometimes millions of dollars on such public statements of their purpose and goals. The truth is that no one in his or her right mind would ever use any portion of the public language of a organization as a guide for his or her behavior. To do so would be (from an organizational point of view) suicidal. It is even more outrageous to suggest (and yet it is often suggested) that such language motivates people to engage in behavior consistent with it.

So how did Henry Ford really get his organization started? He had to have capital. How did he get capital? He sold part of the business. With all the other opportunities that were available, did these people buy Henry Ford's vision? Did they share his dream. No! They did it because he convinced them that giving him their money (by way of investing in the organization) was the best thing they could do to take care of what was important to them. That's what human influence is all about. That's where all organizations begin. Friendships, family, churches, hospitals, universities, that's where they all begin, with somebody creating an aggregation of resources as the best thing to take care of what is important to that individual. Physicians, nurses, volunteers, staff, pharmacists, administrators, patients, patient families, lawyers, legislators, third-party payers. They are all engaged in behavior designed by them to tap into a set of resources and take care of what is important to them. There is no mystery about why we have conflict. The mystery is how we ever get cooperation out of these people.

Now that I have, I hope, effectively demolished the current, very inadequate, theory of organizations and organizational behavior, it is incumbent on me to offer an alternative model. In the next chapter, I will do just that. This model will lead to a discussion of how you can use it to influence, more effectively, the behavior of others and thus the effectiveness of the organizations with which you are associated in terms of serving your values.

CHAPTER FOUR

THE TRUTH
ABOUT ORGANIZATIONS

My alternative organizational model is designed around what I have identified as three functions and three elements of organizations. I use the word "function," not "purpose," "mission," or "objective." This is an important distinction. To illustrate, what does it mean to say that a drinking glass has functions? It means that human beings can use it to take care of some things important to them. Obviously, it can hold liquids, but does it have other possible functions for human beings? A paperweight, a template to draw circles, a weapon, a musical instrument, a listening device. If broken, it could be used as a cutting device. The functions of a drinking glass are limited only by the creativity of the people using it and the physical characteristics of the glass. It is designed for certain functions by somebody, but it can be used for those functions or for many others.

But what about the drinking glass's objectives? What is its mission, vision, strategic plan, philosophy? How does it feel about being picked up? All those questions seem ludicrous when applied to a drinking glass. But that glass, in some sense, has more reality than an organization. It is a physical object. An organization ultimately is a set of neurological pathways in people's brains. People show up at a certain place at a certain time and engage in a certain kind of behavior because of their assumptions about the organization, because of their memories of it. But suppose something happened in the cosmos: A set of rays touches every human on Earth and the consequence of that set of rays touching those people's brains is that all of their knowledge, all of their assumptions, all of their beliefs, all of their memories concerning a particular organization evaporate. The organization no longer exists, because it is only a set of neurological pathways in people's brains. Of course, very different attitudes and views and beliefs about the organization exist in the different brains. But everything about the organization, including its functions, are defined by people and disappear when people are no longer interested or aware.

The first and fundamental function of all organizations is to attract resources. Ford

19

Motor Company ads are not only designed to sell cars. They are also designed to get people to work for Ford Motor Company and to buy stock in Ford Motor Company. They are designed to attract resources for the people in the company. Go back to Henry Ford at the time the company originated. At that point, there is no difference between Henry Ford and the Ford Motor Company. It is an idea in his head. He can talk about the Ford Motor Company at least in potential, about assembly lines and distribution systems. He can paint a picture of something that does not yet exist but will exist if only others will invest in his idea (not share his vision) and invest in him. That's what organizations are fundamentally. They are tools used by human beings to attract resources to themselves. Why did I found the Swarthmore Academy? In order to attract a set of resources to take care of some things that are important to me.

Consider the phrase "investing in a friendship." Did you ever invest in a friendship? You went to a party, you met somebody new, you took down the person's name and phone number. A few days later you overcame your fear of rejection, dialed the phone number, and set up a time to have lunch together. You invested in a friendship. You were trying to add to the aggregation of resources available to you to take care of what is important to you. Did you ever disinvest in a friendship or a job or a marriage? It isn't paying off any more, the aggregation of resources isn't doing what you wanted it to do. Inadequate return on investment. So you invest your time, energy, and resources elsewhere.

The second function of organizations is to transform these resources into something of intrinsic human value. The resources are of no value unless they can be converted into something more immediately useful and satisfying to us. Economists say resources are aggregated so that they can be turned into goods and services. It's deeper than that. The conversion is made in order to satisfy a need. The goods and services are a device to generate and sustain a greater flow of resources. The creation of goods and services is not an end unto itself; it is nothing more than a means. When we take a set of resources and transform it into goods and services, we are doing it specifically to create excess resources that we can gain access to. Yes, we may want to create resources for the client, the patient, the customer, but we want enough left over so that we can tap into them to serve our own values.

And, there is something far more important to us in our organizational affiliations than mere continuity of personal cash flow. Organizations make available what most of us can get only from organizational affiliations and certainly best from organizational affiliations, i.e., ego enhancement. Let me break it down into its constituent elements. Power, security, respect, esteem, status, acceptance, approval, gratitude, appreciation, recognition, success, achievement, autonomy, security, fun, transcendence. The same sorts of value satisfactions Henry Ford was seeking when he created the Ford Motor Company. The rationale for organizations is the attraction of resources so they can be transformed into intrinsic human value satisfactions. They are not about organizational missions, not about organizational visions, not about organizational objectives and goals, not about organizational purposes, not about goods and services. They are, ultimately, mechanisms that people, by their behavior, attempt to tap into to get personal intrinsic value satisfaction. Individuals may have missions, visions, values, objectives and goals, purposes, but organizations cannot.

Publicly, we say something quite different. We point to the client or customer, to the patient, as the reason for the organization. We say that we are all devoted to the same outcomes, we all buy into the same values—patient welfare. That's not what the game is all about. You joined the organization because you perceived that it was the best aggregation of resources available to take care of what is important to you. Not only is that the reason you joined the organization; it also accounts for your behavior 24 hours a day, 7 days a week, in and around that organization. It accounts for the behavior of third-party payers, nurses, pharmacists, volunteers, physicians, patients and their families, lawyers, media representatives, and everyone else who comes into contact with the organization.

Once you accept organizations as being nothing more than artifacts created by human beings to supply them with intrinsic values satisfaction, you discover very interesting things about behavior in organizations. For example, you discover there is no irrational behavior in organizations. Behavior often looks irrational because we compare it to the public language of the organization. If you look at the people in the organization and their behavior, their behavior is totally rational. It makes complete sense from their point of view. If you think that your job is to take these people whose values may not be the same as the values of the organization and harmonize their beliefs with the values of the organization, you are engaged in an absolutely fruitless and highly frustrating pursuit.

This distinction cuts to the heart of your effectiveness. Each person is there to take care of what is important to him or her. This doesn't mean that what is important to each of us is necessarily narrow and selfish and self-centered. What is important may be broad and altruistic. Each of us has, as part of his or her value system, some sense of ethics, morality, justice, and concern for the welfare of others. Professionalism and principle are part of the value system of most people. If you want to get harmony and cooperation and collaboration from people, stop relying on the public language game. Stop assuming we are all here for the same reason. Stop appealing to the mission and vision language of the organization as a way to influence human behavior. It doesn't work for a fundamental reason. It's wrong. If you understand the reason they are there and the reasons they behave as they do, and the reason you are there and the reasons you behave as you do, you may begin to understand the conditions under which they will engage in behaviors that take care of what is important to you.

The third function of organizations, and it follows naturally from the first two functions, is allocation of resources. Once resources have been attracted and transformed into value satisfactions, they are allocated to all of those who are associated with the organization. Organizations are mechanisms for that allocation.

There are three elements that go with these three functions. The first, obviously, is the resources that drive all the functions of an organization. Nobody would be interested in an organization without resources. Without resources there is no organization. We ordinarily think of people as the most important resource—their knowledge, skill, expertise, creativity, enthusiasm—but there are other important resources—supplies, materials, equipment, facilities, etc. I once believed, as most people do, that people are the key organizational resource. But one day, I was having lunch with the chairman of the board of a large energy company and somehow the conversation came around to the resources of his organization. He smiled when I suggested the common wisdom, that people were the company's most valuable resource. "To hell with the people. They're replaceable," he said. "It's the oil in the ground." Two years later, the chairman retired. The people in the organization were euphoric; the oil, as far as I could tell, was indifferent. People are an organizational resource, but they are much more.

People are also the second element in any organization. People play two very different roles in organizations, and traditional organizational theories simply do not recognize, or do not recognize fully, the second role. Being a resource is not people's primary role in organizations. Their primary role is that of seekers after value satisfaction.

We each play the two roles—seeker and resource—simultaneously. I have been on the faculty of the University of Pennsylvania for 27 years. Of those two roles, which dominates my behavior and which one must you understand if you want to influence me? What, from my point of view, am I primarily at that institution? I am a seeker. What is everybody else in that place to me? Potential resources. The common mistake is to see other people in the organization as competitive seekers. My best advice to you is to never see or behave toward anyone as a competitive seeker no matter what their behavior toward you may be. Always see people as potential resources and treat them accordingly. I don't want to fight with you; I want to co-opt you. I don't want to use my time and energy in conflict with you; I want you acting in ways that support what is important to me. I will always attempt to shape the behavior of others as resources, not as competitive seekers. To do that, I have to understand that other people in the organization, in their heads, are seekers. I want them to perceive me as a potential resource. I work to see to it that other people at the University of Pennsylvania perceive me as a resource, not as a competitive seeker. If they perceive me as a resource, we have the potential for cooperation. If they see me as a competitive seeker, they are likely to come in conflict with me.

The third element of an organization brings this discussion full circle. At any given time, each organization has limited resources. Further, at any given time, the set of demands on those resources will tend to exceed the supply of the resources. People, as seekers (at least most Americans), are insatiable in their demands for value satisfaction. No matter how much you give people, they are very likely to ask for more. Have your employees ever come to you and said they are being paid more than they're worth? How about patients with third-party payer coverage? Do they say that quality is too high and cost too low and that the ratio should be changed? When was the last time your children came to you and told you they had tapped you enough, and told you that it's payback time for them?

If these two propositions are valid—all organizations have limited resources and the demands on those resources tend to exceed the supply of those resources—we need operational priorities within the organization—the third element of this model of organization. What we need is an adjudicatory mechanism. All organizations have to have some mechanism by which the limited resources, the limited value satisfactions, are allocated across greater or even unlimited demands. We have resources (potential value satisfactions), we have seekers (human beings looking for value satisfaction), and we need something to determine who is going to get what.

Let's look at that first human organization, some 75,000 years ago. As far as we know, the first human beings formed organizations, clans, kinship units, families for purposes of safety and security. And when one joins an organization, you can't do what you want, when you want, where you want, how you want. When you are in a group to get the security, the sense of survival, the protection of an organization, pragmatically, you have to look to the interests of others.

Let's say someone was lucky enough to bring down a wild pig and drags it back to camp. Everybody comes out of the cave and forms a circle around the pig, pointing and shouting, "resource, resource." But there isn't enough pig to go around, and some parts of the pig are thought to be better than other parts of the pig. So we have the first resource allocation problem in the history of humankind. At that point, someone invented what has become the universal, indeed the ubiquitous, adjudicatory mechanism. Power! Not authority, not hierarchy, not the chief but power. Even back then there was, no doubt, a distribution of power, negotiation going on.

The word may stick in your throat, because the media, television in particular, tend to paint only the coercive, negative, excessive side of power. Power is much broader than that. Power is nothing more than one's ability to tap into organizational resources to serve one's own values. It takes many manifestations, many forms, and it is the third and final element of organizational life.

We each want more power. Cooperation, collaboration, and synergy are available to you commensurately with the power you have in the organization. You and I may have some illusion of direct control over a tiny piece of organizational resources, but, for the most part, tapping into the resources of an organization means influencing the behavior of people—board members, chiefs, physicians, secretaries, nurses, volunteers, administrators, patients, patients' families, lawyers, media, legislators, and so on. What we want out of the organization in terms of intrinsic value satisfaction is ultimately available only in the behavior of those people. If we don't know how to shape the patterns of our own behavior, more often than not we will end up in all sorts of dysfunctional and counterproductive conflicts. If we do control our own behavior and if we are able to stimulate certain patterns of it in others, by definition, we have power. We have enhanced our ability to influence the patterns of behavior of the people who allocate the resources that serve our values.

CHAPTER FIVE

VALUES AND HOW THEY GET SERVED

Why do people in organizations use public language—mission statements, vision statements, etc.? One, it's an easy and safe behavior to engage in. Two, it has a certain romance to it. Three, it insulates the people who create it from the responsibility for executing it. It's a buffer. Four, it has now become an expectation. Many things get done in organizations because of habit or tradition, because they "are supposed to be done." If you do not create mission statements and vision statements, you're not in the flow of things. Total quality management is, again, a good example. There isn't anything that I have seen in TQM that hasn't been around for 25 or 30 years or even longer. But we have to have something new on the scene that we all say we are doing.

Let me offer you an example from my experience. When parents of prospective students call the Swarthmore Academy to learn more about what it does, we give them a brochure that gives the objectives, goals, mission, and values of the Swarthmore Academy. A brochure that I wrote. I don't think the faculty, staff, students, and parents read my brochure each morning in order to know what to do that day. Some of them have never read it. Some of them never will read it. They are not there to take care of what is important to me, and they are not there to serve the "mission of the organization." They are there to take care what is important to them. I have to understand that if I want to influence their behavior.

How many of you have the basic Equal Employment Opportunity objective stated somewhere in your organizational documents? Your organization is an affirmative action employer and does not discriminate on the basis of age, gender, race, or national origin. Is that statement a deep and abiding value commitment of the chairman of the board? Do employees know that it is intended as a guide for their behavior? Do they know what happens if they engage in behavior supportive of the statement? Do they know what happens if they ignore it? Do they know what happens if they engage in behavior contrary to it? The answer in all cases is almost certainly "no." Then why make the statement? Someone from the Equal Employment Opportunity Commission arrives, takes some time and energy away from you, and threatens to cut off some set of resources to you if you don't put the statement on a piece of paper. Often, it is no more complicated than that. It doesn't mean you have to do anything that is consistent with the statement. You put it on the piece of paper so that you are able to show it to somebody.

Some of these verbal exercises are nothing more than self-aggrandizement. A CEO I have done some work for has 10 objectives for his organization every year. On January 1, every department in the organization has 10 objectives for the new year. They are so general, so vague, they couldn't influence anybody's behavior. But they make him feel good. You cannot walk into a bathroom of that organization without seeing his statement of 10 objectives. Do those statements influence behavior? Yes. Everyone in the organization ridicules the statements whenever they don't think the CEO is around. Some statements are made to keep representatives of federal agencies at bay. Some are made as acts of self-aggrandizement. Others are made to provide eye wash for investors or for the board or for anyone else who is demanding some statement of what the organization is all about. They are nothing more than the product of behaviors designed to take care of something important to the people who create the language. What is problematic about them is that some chief executive officers and other managers actually believe that issuing them will somehow alter patterns of behavior in some positive way. They seem to believe that such statements guide or motivate. They don't, and they won't.

In order to reinforce this point, try the following experiment. Pretend that the public language of your organization, in terms of mission statements, vision statements, etc., represents the most important values in your life. That you are now going to engage in patterns of behavior that are totally devoted to, for instance, "patient welfare." What will happen? You will be gone from the organization. Some of the behaviors that you will engage in will tread on the toes of powerful people in the organization, and they won't like it. They will use their power to make sure you don't engage in any more of those behaviors.

Let me give an example. Nurses, in their professional socialization in nursing school, are taught patient welfare as their primary professional value. They are told that they are supposed to report anyone, including physicians, who engages in behavior that, in any way, threatens patient welfare. Report it, challenge it, do something about it. Nurse compliance with that value has been tested. In one experiment, less than 15 percent of the nurses who believe a doctor had instructed them to do something threatening to the patient reported it to anyone; 85 percent of the nurses attempted to do as instructed. Why did so many nurses fail to follow through on that professional value? They would very likely have had to put themselves at serious risk in their profession to engage in behavior consistent with that piece of public language. Job, career, acceptance, approval, autonomy, security, welfare, welfare of their families—all would probably have been at risk, or at least that is what many of them perceived.

So what is the point of public language? Should we abandon it? No—not at all. It can be useful, and, in any case, others will expect it of you. To abandon it might put you and your values at risk. Sometimes it can even be fun to use. Let's suppose I go to a dinner party that's a disaster. I make for the door as early as I possibly can, but the hostess catches me at the door and asks if I had a good time. I don't say that the party was a world class flop. I dig for some public language, preferably with a little ambiguity, and say, "actually this is one of the more enjoyable experiences of my life." I am referring to the fact that I am leaving, and she thinks I am talking about her party. Both of our needs are satisfied, and there is no hurt. That is a desirable (albeit somewhat trivial) outcome of the use of public language.

To do our jobs, we often perceive that we have to violate the policies, rules, and regulations of the organization. All policies, rules, and regulations were created by some human being or some group of human beings to take care of something important to them. A lead article in the *New York Times* in 1990 reported on an interview with three principals of New York City high schools. The principals were incredibly honest. They said what everybody in the system knows. They can't educate kids unless they circumvent the rules, regulations, and policies of the New York City School System. It is still easy to get sucked back into the paradigm of organizations that says they are about missions, vision, objectives, goals, patient welfare, community health care, and so on. They are not. They are about the individual personal agendas of the human beings who engage in their value-directed behaviors in and around organizations. If people in organizations are to be influenced, it will have to be in terms of those agendas and not in terms of the public statements of the organization.

There are three ways you can have your values served. You can have your values served by coincidence. Somebody engages in behavior designed by them to take care of something important to them, and your values are served by chance, perhaps without your knowledge. For example, somebody at the American College of Physician Executives chooses the location for a seminar at which I will be faculty. I have no voice in the choice, but it is a very pleasant environment in which to give a seminar. My values are served by the behavior of that ACPE staff person. I doubt seriously that the person had my values in mind when the location was chosen. He or she was taking care of something that was important to him or her. My satisfaction is coincidental. The second way in which we can get our values served is that somebody who has power values serving some of our values. Patients often have their values served in hospitals not because they have power but because many physicians, nurses, and other people in hospitals value giving good patient care. It enhances their self-esteem, fulfills their sense of professional obligation and makes them feel good about themselves. The newborn infant tends to get its values served initially because somebody who has power values serving at least some of the infant's values. One of the reasons many children don't like school is that they don't have much power to tap into the school's resources. But some students do get their values served in schools, because there are many principals and teachers who value serving the students' values; they are genuinely concerned about the children's welfare.

The third way of getting your values served is through the personal use of power. My assumption is that that is your preference. It certainly is mine. I do not want to depend upon either chance or largesse to have my values served.

One way to understand power is to contrast it with authority. They are quite different things. Power is the ability to use your behavior to tap into the resources of an organization and get your values served. Authority, on the other hand, is nothing more than an organizational privilege extended to you by someone in the organization to engage in certain behaviors in the expectation of being supported in those behaviors. It's not a right. It is a privilege. It's temporary. It's fragile and can disappear in an instant. It's expensive. Every increase in authority is accompanied by an increase in responsibility, and the latter almost always outruns the former in magnitude. The all too frequently experienced gap between one's authority and one's responsibility has to be filled with one's power.

People often believe that if they only have more authority, everything will be fine. They feel that they have too much responsibility without commensurate authority. And when additional authority is finally granted, it seems always to be accompanied by additional responsibility. Few ever believe that they have enough authority to execute their responsibilities. More responsibility is the cost of authority. The reason is simple. When the same person assigns both authority and responsibility, they are more inclined to give responsibility, less inclined to give authority. Once again, one fills the gap between authority and responsibility with power.

It is, of course, possible to have enormous authority and no power. There are people at the top of organizations with maximum authority and little or no power because they are weak-willed and indecisive. All the people below them in the organization do as they please. It is also possible to have zero authority and enormous power. If you are employed in a hospital for which there are some substantial donors, you will understand. People who give megabucks to the organization aren't on the organizational chart. They have zero authority. But when they and theirs come to the hospital for treatment, they are not treated like everybody else. They receive special treatment because someone with power in the organization wants to influence their behavior so that these donors may continue to be resources (or at least not offend them and eliminate the possibility of a future flow of resources).

Don't seek authority in an organization, focus on power. Authority is fragile, temporary, and limited. It is always accompanied by responsibility, accountability. Power has unlimited potential and no cost in terms of accountability. It has its own cost, but it doesn't cost in terms of added responsibility and accountability. A curious thing about power is that the more you get, the more people want to heap authority on you. You have demonstrated the ability to influence behavior to get your values served, and others want to use you for that power. You are a potential resource to take care of what is important to them. An example will illustrate the concept.

Magic Johnson of the Los Angeles Lakers played basketball. He put the ball through the hoop, made assists, rebounds. He demonstrated charismatic leadership. Yet where was he on the organizational chart? How much authority did he have? Zero. Who had authority over Magic Johnson, to whom did Magic Johnson report in the organizational chart? Coach Mike Dunleavy. Yet when there was a dispute between Magic Johnson and the coach of the Los Angeles Lakers, it is Magic Johnson who had the power. If that is unclear in your mind, you may wish to interview the former coach of the Los Angeles Lakers whom Magic had fired. Magic is someone without authority who had a great deal of power.

What was the ultimate basis of Magic Johnson's power? Skill? Charisma? Performance? His ability to generate income, cash flow, TV receipts? In general to attract resources to the organization? It is not quite any of those. None of these is either necessary or sufficient for power. Magic is unique, but that isn't necessary or sufficient for power. He affected the performance of the organization, brought prestige to the club and the owner, but those aren't necessary or sufficient for the acquisition of power. Magic Johnson was a resource of great magnitude to the Los Angeles Lakers, but his power resided in the perceptions of certain key figures. Others, most notably those above him in the organization chart, including the owner of the club, perceived that the resource called Magic Johnson would be lost to them unless they behaved in certain ways. Magic was able to influence that behavior because he was able to put certain perceptions in others' heads.

Perceptions are personal, fragile, subjective, arbitrary, and idiosyncratic, but fortunately they are also infinitely malleable. Suppose everything said about Magic Johnson was true but the owner did not believe it. Then Magic would have no power with him. Suppose everything said about Magic Johnson is false, but the owner believed it to be true. Then, Magic Johnson has substantial potential (but only potential) power. It is only potential because the owner not only has to believe that Magic Johnson is an indispensable resource, scores points, and brings glory to the owner and to his team, but also has to perceive that unless he (the owner) engages in quite specific behaviors, Magic Johnson will no longer be available to him. Many people make the mistake of believing that if they just keep their noses to the grindstone, they will be rewarded. If you keep your nose to the grindstone, you will end up with a bloody nose. If you are counting on your value as a resource to influence then you have to put the perception in the other person's head that, unless he or she engages in certain behaviors, you, as a resource, won't be available. Power is the ability, directly or indirectly, to put quite specific perceptions into another person's head.

It is also critical to remember that all behavior is essentially prospective. All behavior is in anticipation that it is going to deliver something for us. What I have to do, through my behavior, is put a perception in your head that your values will best be served if you engage in a certain behavior. That is the essence of power. I have to shape the data fragments of my behavior so that you end up with that neurological connection in your head. If you do, I get the behavior I want. If you don't, I don't get the behavior I want. Magic Johnson had some advantages—natural ability and the concentrated effort he has put into what he does—but that is neither necessary nor sufficient for power. If the owner thought that Magic Johnson was a committed player who would always give his best for the Los Angeles Lakers and for professional basketball no matter what the owner does, Magic Johnson has no power. It doesn't matter how good he is or what contribution he makes or how he is perceived as long as the owner doesn't perceive that he (the owner) has to engage in certain behaviors to maintain Magic as a resource.

There is probably no human activity monitored more meticulously than professional sports. The behavior of every single athlete is analyzed and reanalyzed and documented and categorized. Yet even in this most carefully monitored human activity, there is subjectivity. The statistics say one thing, subjective perceptions of fans and owners say another. It may serve the values of the owner to have lunch

Values and How They Get Served

every Thursday with his sports legend, even though the player's statistics are a mere shadow of what they once were. It's worth a million dollars a year so that the player is still in the limelight and the owner is still the player's buddy. Power is perception. And, perceptions are subjective, personal, fragile, arbitrary, idiosyncratic, and infinitely malleable.

How much more or less subjective is your world or mine? Each organization consists of a group of people working out their value agendas, attempting to tap into resources by influencing the behavior of other people in the organization. We have been brought up to believe that influence has to do with right, truth, reason, argument, logic, evidence, fact, quality, substance, and the like, but it doesn't. Those are admirable values to have, but we live in a world of data fragments, subjective impressions, and idiosyncratic judgments. People in communications research have told me that the average American adult is confronted on a daily basis with between 350 and 700 messages trying to influence his or her behavior. I have heard numbers as high as 1,800 for such messages. Every phone call, memo, billboard, bulletin board, ad, commercial, meeting, informal discussion, and seminar is jammed with data fragments designed to influence us.

The capacity for technology to dump messages on us is increasing (electronic mail, electronic voice mail), but the number of hours in the day hasn't increased. Our capacity for processing information in our brains hasn't increased. We have had to build both subconscious and conscious barriers inside of our brains, filters or screens that allow some things through but keep most things out. Usually, we are not consciously aware of the operation of these filtration systems in our brains. Think of the process by which you sort your mail, at home or in the office. You pick up a piece of mail and, in less than a second, you can determine what to do with it. In less than a second, you pick up a whole series of data fragments from that piece of mail. Where it came from. How much postage is on it and how the postage was placed on it. How it was addressed—handwritten, individually typed, or a computer-generated label. Whether it says "personal and confidential," even if it is addressed to "occupant."

Those who wish to influence your behavior in your processing of your mail also have systems. You pick up a piece of mail with an innocuous return address. It has a third-class bulk indicia in the right hand corner, but your name and address appear inside of the window. It also shows the words, "Pay to the order of." It turns out that some of the people who process product rebate checks know that many people discard such mail unopened because they perceive it as a gimmick used by direct mail marketers. So they are now sending rebate checks the same way in anticipation that the checks will be discarded. There are many such people trying to influence our behavior. They are paid to figure out how to get through our filters and get us to do what they want us to do. But they do not always succeed, even when they may have something of great value to bring to our attention. So you and I, as we filter through third-class mail, doubtless throw things out that, if we paid more conscious attention to them, would have influenced our behavior and possibly even served our values. We throw out the good with the bad. We have to because of the volume of data fragments competing for our attention.

What does this have to do with human influence? It tells us that when we are trying to influence people, we are only a few of those hundreds of data fragments competing for others' behavior. It tells us that if we don't design, more consciously, more deliberatively, the data fragments of our own behavior, we will never get through their filters. If we don't get through their filters, it doesn't matter how good our ideas are. It doesn't matter how much value satisfaction it would deliver to them if only they would listen to us. The only thing that counts is whether it will get through their filters. And everyone's filtration system is becoming more arbitrary, more automatic, and quicker. We cannot count on truth or right or reasonableness or evidence or objectivity. We cannot count on quality or substance to aid us in our attempts at human influence.

Let's take an example from health care—and toys. Hospitals and toy companies face a similar challenge in their marketing, in their efforts to influence people. The consumer and the purchaser are different agents. The toy companies have decided to go after the consumer, primarily through Saturday morning cartoons. There is a weakness when you go to the consumer, however. You must influence the consumer so powerfully that the consumer becomes the sales agent to influence the purchaser. There is an additional link in the chain of influence. In health care, the purchaser and the consumer are not only different agents, they have opposing agendas. The consumer wants high-quality, state-of-the-art care. The purchaser wants high quality, but is more concerned with price and need. But the consumer of health care services is largely incompetent to judge the quality of service. Most will judge the hospital experience on the basis of food, housekeeping, whether the wheels squeak on the carts, how quickly staff answers the call button, how easy it is to sleep, the decor, etc. So hospitals put resources into cosmetics, not because it will increase the quality of health care but because it will affect the consumer's perception and, therefore, what he or she says about the hospital to other people. Those resources, siphoned off in support of these superficialities, are likely to be taken away from what is needed to support the quality of health care. All of us, if we wish to influence human behavior, are increasingly required to deal with cosmetics,

Values and How They Get Served

superficialities. If we don't package our messages well, they won't get through the filters. If they don't get through the filters, they are lost and useless.

So each of us receives data fragments, and we do not have the time to give conscious consideration to all the messages competing for our behavior. We make snap decisions based on a fragment here and a fragment there. Of course, we are also sending out data fragments, and others are reacting to them in just this way. We are competing, because of the hundreds if not thousands of data fragments that are being thrown at those people whom we wish to influence on a daily basis. If we are going to increase our power, we will have to be more precisely targeted with our messages. There is no magic. There can be no guarantees. It is a matter of deliberately constructing our data fragments to increase the probability that they will get through with the intended effect. There is too much complexity, too much fragility in the modern world to assume that we can always shape the data fragments of our behavior to put what we want in others' heads. But, with effort, we can do it more often and more effectively.

There is one more piece of public language that I want to explore before completing this discussion—the concept of organizational problems. My position is that the organization cannot possibly have problems. An organizational problem would be a deviation from organizational objectives, but organizations don't have objectives. There are pseudo-problems in organizations. At a staff meeting, somebody bemoans malpractice insurance, court cases, new legislative incentives, DRGs, whatever. Like a Greek chorus the whole group joins in. But, by the end of the meeting, nobody has done anything about the alleged problem except agonized over it. Each leaves the meeting and goes back to what is functionally, operationally important to each. The problem that has no impact on behavior isn't a problem.

Not only are there no organizational problems; there also are no shared problems. That statement is contrary to our enculturation, but it's true. The statement that there is a shared problem is, in fact, nothing more than a series of data fragments sent to influence the behavior of others. But even when the boss walks in and says, "We have a problem," it's not a shared problem. You may now have a problem but it's not the boss's problem. Your problem is dealing **with** the boss.

Another example will expose the folly of the shared problem notion. You walk into a staff meeting with the solution to the alleged organizational problem. You have thought about it and come up with this elegant solution. You present it to your colleagues with eloquence and excitement, even though it means their budgets will be cut 15 percent and some of their staff will have to be laid off. You are met with a lot of hostility. Your position is that sacrifices have to be made for the "good of the organization. We are all in this together, aren't we." No! They are processing the data fragments of your behavior and asking themselves what it has to do with them and their values.

What does the phrase, "Good for the organization," mean? It has no meaning outside of good for the individual using the phrase. Have you noticed that your solutions to "organizational problems" tend to serve your values? Did you think that is just a happy coincidence? We play these games in our heads because we have been taught to, and they reduce our effectiveness. They feel good, but they certainly don't make us more powerful. There may be some phenomenon in the external world that you perceive as a threat to your values and that I perceive as a threat to my values, but that doesn't mean we have a shared problem. How we perceive that the phenomenon threatens our values, and what we are each willing to do to serve our individual, personal values, might be quite different.

How do we get cooperation from people, if it isn't through shared problems? Is it through shared values? Be careful with that answer; that is the origin of the notion of organizational culture. The concept is about 15 years old in broad usage, and there is a great deal of literature to describe it and tout it. The notion of an organizational culture is very dangerous. Organizational theorists apparently used up all of sociology in their publications and were looking for new bottles for their old wine. They stumbled across anthropology, and now we hear about organizational values, organizational rituals, organizational taboos, organizational language. It is a phrase out of cultural anthropology, inappropriately applied. It is the larger culture of which you and I are a part that shapes our fundamental values between birth and about age seven. It is appropriate to talk about something called cultural values. But as soon as one applies the term to organizations, one has assumed that the organization not only has values but also shapes the values of others. Many people argue that if only we can bring people together, if only we can get shared values, shared visions, and get them to buy into the values of the organization, cooperation will follow. All of this regrettable public language is reinforced by this misapplication of cultural anthropology.

Organizations don't have values, and I assure you that they are not going to reshape peoples values. We continue to insist that we can bring people together on values and get cooperation. But it's not true, and even if it were possible to change people's values, the results might not be agreeable. The most vicious behavior conceivable has been reserved, historically, for situations wherein people have been closest in values. Often in civil wars, one can barely tell the difference between the combatants. Religious wars, particularly intra-religious wars, are another example. There is something about people just like us that we can really hate. Even when we do have values similar to those of others, we will, as they will, interpret them in our own idiosyncratic ways, and those values will take a certain priority among our values that will be specific for each of us. It is not shared values that bring people together into cooperative relationships. And, in any case, you are not going to change the values of other adults in your organization.

We often seem to believe that life will be better if we have people around us who share our values. I am not particularly interested in being surrounded by people who supposedly share my values. I want to be surrounded by people who are willing to engage in behavior that serves my values. That is quite a different thing. The former almost routinely leads to conflict, because we assume that similarity of values automatically facilitates cooperation. The latter is a building block for cooperation because, contrary to our enculturation, conflict and cooperation are not primarily a function of values and philosophies and ideologies. Conflict and cooperation are both based in behaviors and perceptions, not in ideology. Until you engage in a behavior that I perceive threatens my values and I engage in a counterbehavior that you perceive as threatening your values, there is no conflict. People of opposite ideologies can come together and cooperate. When they do, we say they make for strange bedfellows. Understand that differences, or even opposition, in values do not necessarily lead to behaviors and perceptions that produce conflict. Indeed, potential conflicts can be turned into cooperation, collaboration, and synergy as long as we recognize the likely differences in values, acknowledge the power that others have, and then, sensitive to their interests, find behaviors for them that we bring them to perceive will best serve their values.

CHAPTER SIX

SEARCHING FOR EFFECTIVE BEHAVIORS

While the process of designing an organizational mission statement, as opposed to the statement itself, could be useful, I don't think it often is. The statement is a **tool** (not necessarily a representation) of the values of those with the greatest power in the organization. If somebody suggested a participative process for the creation of a mission statement and the patterns of behavior in the organization are open, it could have some process value for the people involved with it. But too many claims are made about the process value of getting people in the organization involved in the activity of creating a mission statement. Each person who gets involved in that process is waiting to see whether or not the rewards and punishments, the allocation of resources, will actually bear any resemblance to what it was they got excited about, if they got excited about it in the first place. What they know is that it often won't.

I did some work for the New York Stock Exchange several years ago. The CEO and other executives of the New York Stock Exchange spent an enormous amount of organizational resource getting everyone, at all managerial levels, involved in determinations of what values, principles, and ethical guidelines the Stock Exchange was going to have. People went on retreats and came back with not only what these things were but presumably what they meant to everyone. What is critical is whether the words generated by such processes actually got specific people engaged in specific patterns of behavior that are necessarily consistent with, or supportive of, or furthering the language that an enormous amount of New York Stock Exchange resources went into creating. Usually that final stage is never achieved. When the former CEO left, the new director of the New York Stock Exchange may or may not have decided to pay attention to all those things his predecessor did. I suppose it's a benign exercise to undertake from time to time, but the return in terms of alterations in patterns of behavior probably makes it less than an effective way to use organizational resources.

Let me contrast that with behavior that I think is more likely to be lasting and to show results. It is essential for you to have an explicit notion of what you would like to see your particular unit or the organization as a whole look like, of how you would make measurable progress toward that goal. Most people don't do that, because they are not really interested in developing new initiatives. If you are concerned about that future view, you should get very explicit, concrete, measurable, and observable about it. What would an ideal department, division, unit, hospital, PPO or HMO look like?

Whether or not you choose to share that personal vision or mission is very much an issue of implementation. If you share the idea, you may scare people. You may warn people who don't want that kind of an organization and give them that much more time to prepare against it. I have a personal mission for Swarthmore Academy. I share pieces of my vision on occasion with the faculty. I don't share with the faculty if I don't think it is the right place or the right time. Likewise, I have a sense in my head of the direction I want the division at the University of Pennsylvania that I chair to pursue. I am not at all confident that sharing my mission or vision or asking others for their missions or visions is a particularly useful way to move the organization in the direction that I have in mind. What I want is patterns of behavior in support of my values that people come to perceive are best for what is important to them. I am not concerned with whether they "buy" my values or mission (whatever that means). I want them engaged in behavior that is sympathetic to, and in support of, outcomes that are important to me and consistent with my values.

On balance, then, the production of mission and other public statements is not a particularly good investment of resources to alter patterns of behavior. I am not saying that we should never think these organizational matters through. There are people who, for their own reasons, want a sense of the whole organization, a sense of where it's going. You may want to give that to them. But there many people who don't. When I was a graduate student at Cornell in the early 1960s, everybody was talking about participative management, the democratic work place, and so on. Then, in the mid-1960s, data started coming in from organizations that showed there were many people in organizations who did not want to participate at all. They wanted to know what behavior was desired and what was in it for them to comply with it. It is still true of a good many people. Some people don't want to participate, some people don't want to vote, some people don't want to take responsibility for outcomes. They want a relatively narrow, structured world. So, where it is effective to share, do so, and where it isn't, don't. But don't assume that there is some magical formula out there for getting everybody to buy into your (not the organization's) vision or mission.

Searching for Effective Behaviors

Given this view of organizations, why don't we have anarchy, chaos? Two reasons. First is our concern for others' welfare, our principles of justice, mercy, ethics, obligation, morality, and professionalism. These notions are, thankfully, built into the value systems of most of us. We do have a sense of concern for the welfare of others, some sense of responsibility to others in the organization, to patients, nursing staff, colleagues, and subordinates. Second, we have, at some level, been wise enough to understand the potential for chaos and have worked out multiple arrangements that allow people with very different values and very different agendas to come together and cooperate. That is what a money exchange system is all about. I don't have to go into a store and share values with the person behind the counter. They have their values, and I have mine. We have created an exchange system. I give the person something that serves his or her values; he or she gives me something that serves my values. We don't have to have a common cause or shared visions or anything else shared, except an understanding of the individual, personal benefits of this convention for exchange.

Do we have to have shared values in order for these techniques to work? No. They are conventions and principles that we all accept. Most of the time, people will, in fact, abide by convention, because each sees it in his or her best interests to do so. I stop complete strangers in the street and ask them for the time of day. We don't have to have a meeting of minds around common values. It is a convention, and most of the time people will try to accommodate me because of a whole series of socialization processes that they have been through and understandings that we have. We have many such conventions that allow individuals with differing values to pursue those values cooperatively, without isolation, chaos, or conflict with others.

How does the coach of a Superbowl-bound team get the behavior that he wants out of the members of that team? He might assume that every member of the team wants to win the Superbowl. Therefore, he will have no problem getting the behavior patterns he wants from them. I don't think so. Winning the Superbowl for each of them is a means toward personal value satisfaction. Some players want the victory for the glory. Some want it for the cash. Others want it for the prestige, to prove something to themselves, for pride. Some of them want it for the "hotdogging" they can do. The coach has to understand the different motivations and the intensities that people have in their desire to win the Superbowl. He cannot assume that long rivalries or personality difficulties or insecurities or old wars are going to disappear among his players simply because they all say they want to win the Superbowl.

Outside of generally accepted principles of behavior and the conventions that we have established, we avoid chaos by finding those ways of doing things, allocating resources in which multiple individuals are served. I have to find those behaviors on your part that you can come to perceive will take care of what is important to you and that will simultaneously take care of what is important to me. The more of those behaviors we can deliberately and consciously find beyond the conventions that we use, the more we can take potential conflict and turn it into cooperation.

Later in this book, I will be developing a model for influencing human behavior that can be used both positively and negatively. My experience at the University of Pennsylvania illustrates both approaches. I attempt to put the perception in the minds of people at the University that I am a valuable resource both actually and potentially. I do that by, among other things, attracting significant resources to my school. I engage in behaviors I am not required to engage in that bring in significant revenues. A few years ago, some of my colleagues somehow got a perception in their heads that was not to my advantage. To wit, that Charles Dwyer is a nice guy and is going to continue to do this. They thought ours was not a contingent, conditional, dependent relationship. When I asked them for some modest help for one of my students and they said "no," I turned off the faucet. Now they understood. I would be a source of value satisfaction to them to the extent that they were available as a source of value satisfaction to me. If they break what I regarded as an implicit contract, they will no longer see these resources flowing to them through me.

It is critical for people to understand the exact nature of that arrangement. In "High Noon," Gary Cooper, the sheriff of the town, cleaned the town up and everybody was indebted to him. Presumably, he had all kinds of chits built up, but he had announced his intention to marry Grace Kelly and resign as sheriff. In the movie, he was going to leave the next day. The villain who had terrorized the town and whom Cooper had sent to prison was returning to town, and several of his men were waiting for him at the train station. All of them were coming to get Cooper. Cooper went to three different sources to collect his chits. The men at the bar who helped him once before laugh him out of the bar. His best friend hides and won't even see him. The honest folks in town have the deepest debt to him, because he is the one who made it possible for them to walk the streets in safety. They conclude that it would be best if he left town. Why? He made a fatal error in his attempt to influence human behavior. The next day, he would no longer be a continuing source of chits to them. After tomorrow, he would no longer be a source of potential value satisfaction to them. And so, for this and other reasons, his approaches didn't work.

One of the things I have to be clearly aware of, when I get close to retirement and let people know I am retiring from the University of Pennsylvania, is that it won't matter how many chits I have built up. It is not just a matter of paying me back, which some people will do out of a sense of equity. It is that I will no longer be seen as a source of continuing value satisfaction to many of my colleagues and the chits I have built up will be discounted.

So one of the ways to influence people is to have them perceive a transaction is taking place. You give to them, they give to you. Another way, one that has nothing to do with transactions, is simply for me to act as a friend to you and point out to you a whole series of value satisfactions that will flow to you if you engage in a certain behaviors. That series of value satisfaction may have nothing whatsoever to do with me. I am not giving you anything, I am simply bringing you to perceive that, if you engage in a certain behavior, the flow to you is very likely. Whatever technique I use, I put a perception in your head that if you engage in certain behavior, your values will be served best. I may or may not be the one to serve your values. They may be served by somebody else or by circumstance. If you fail to engage in this behavior, I want you to perceive that you will lose an opportunity to gain value satisfaction in your life. Therefore, it is in your interest to engage in this behavior. If I am successful in this approach, you will engage in behavior I want you to engage in not because I am going to give you something if you do, not because I am going to take something away from you if you don't, but because you now perceive that if you don't engage in the behavior, there may be some loss of opportunity for you.

There is at least the vague possibility of threat with this approach to influence. When I deal with subordinates, no matter how positive I am in my behavior toward them in my attempt to influence them, they are always aware of our relative positions. They are aware of what I might do if they don't engage in the behavior I want. I don't necessarily want to reinforce that view, but I'm not going to spend a lot of time and energy trying to eliminate it. I don't want it to dominate my reputation, but I don't mind people believing that there could be negative consequences if they fail to engage in the behavior that I want. Sometimes, I will deliberately put that thought in their minds, but not often, for reasons I will explain later.

Values are at the heart of all behavior. In order to influence another person's behavior, you have to know and understand their values. As indicated earlier, all of these fundamental values are formed in our childhoods. Notions of right and wrong, good and bad, satisfaction and dissatisfaction, happiness and unhappiness. To use this concept of values to understand and influence behavior, I have to expand it to include what I would call hard-wired, genetically determined, DNA-based values.

The Shifting Sources of Power and Influence

We do not come into the world neutral. We come in with needs and wants, desires, predilections, preferences. We want food. To be warm and dry, comfortable. The infant wants love. Behaviorally, that means physical contact of a certain kind. To be held, to be touched, to be cuddled. We want at least one other thing—to be amused. Our senses have a certain structure to them, and there are certain stimuli that are immediately satisfying. Certain sights, colors, touches. As soon as we have one of those pleasant experiences, we don't have to interpret it. We just have to feel it to want it repeated.

Then the culture puts an overlay of values in us—our acquired values. That is part of what we mean by culture and that is why I object to the notion of "organizational culture." Cultural values are held by and spread through individuals. Organizational culture is nothing more than patterns of behavioral acquiescence to power, but we pretend it is something else. Organizations do have profiles, characteristics. I can empirically distinguish IBM from Apple Computer in terms of what we are loosely calling its organizational culture. But I don't think it is a matter of mindset. I don't think it is a substantial difference in the values of the people. It is a matter of selecting people into those organizations whose individual patterns of behavior are likely to accommodate to the people who have power in those organizations. If people leave IBM and go to Apple, it's not because they are seeking a change of values. Their values at IBM are going to be the same values at Apple. They are looking for a set of resources that they believe will better serve their values than the way those values are being served at IBM.

Indeed, we count on stability and continuity in people's values systems. What we know from studies of value development is that our intrinsic values—senses of security and autonomy, acceptance and approval, appreciation, gratitude, recognition, success, achievement, self-esteem, fun, etc.—are put in our heads between birth and age seven. We don't have a concept of security until we have experienced insecurity. We then say we want some permanence, some predictability, some control over our world. Our values may change in priority or intensity during our lives depending upon the environment we are in, but they are not going to change in content. That's what gives the lie to the notion of organizational values, of getting people to buy into organizational values. It is arrogant and absurd to think that a CEO can send out a few data fragments and, as a consequence, make some fundamental alteration in anyone's set of intrinsic values. We spend our entire lives protecting and enhancing the fundamental set of value satisfactions that were put into our heads between birth and age seven. Our behavior in organizations is designed either to protect our self-esteem, security, autonomy, appreciation, gratitude, success, or achievement or to provide an increase in our satisfaction of these values.

We are born with something in addition to hard-wired values. We are also born with hard-wired behaviors. There are certain things you can do when you are born that you don't have to learn. You can breath, suck, swallow, sleep, eliminate wastes, cry, dilate the pupils of your eyes, blink, turn your head, grasp, move your arms and legs. It is similar to the boot-up program in a personal computer. There's not much there, but it's enough to get things started. What we don't appear to have at birth, however, is knowledge of possible connections between our hard-wired behaviors and our hard-wired values. Fortunately for us, by accident (not by trial and error) we begin almost at once to make some of those connections. The infant in a crib doesn't have the vaguest idea of what to do about discomfort or even that anything can be done about it. The infant may, quite naturally, start to flail about, moving its arms and legs. Coincidentally, that moves its trunk and the infant is more comfortable. A neurological memory trace inside the infant's brain connects the behavior with the value satisfaction. The next time it is uncomfortable, the response will come more quickly and efficiently.

Through repeated experience, the infant, and then the child, adolescent, and adult, refine those patterns. We spend our lives refining connections between behavior and value satisfaction. We make linkages in our brain between what is important to us and the behaviors that gain them for us. Another thing we stumble upon by accident is that certain of our behaviors allow us to influence other people whose behavior, in turn, serves our values. Most of what an infant values, requires the cooperation of someone else for satisfaction. At first, the infant has no control over whether people give it that satisfaction. But one day in the first few weeks of life, the infant engages in a behavior and immediately thereafter gets something that it wants. That behavior in this, as in most cultures, is crying. Management technique number one. There are some people in every organization whose managerial repertoire has not increased significantly since their birth. When they want something, they cry, moan, complain, make noise. If others cooperate, it works. Every day in our lives, we reward people who engage in behavior that irritates us and thus reinforce their behavior patterns. It would be more effective, of course, not to reward them, but it could be costly. If there is a history of rewards, they will probably persist for a while in the undesired behavior. They may even escalate the behavior for a while because that is one of their ways of getting what they want. Eventually, if not rewarded and reinforced, the behavior will cease because it is no longer working and, in their perception, is an ineffective way to use their time and energy.

So what is power? It is your repertoire of such behaviors. Each of us has a repertoire of both direct and indirect behaviors. The infant's behaviors are initially direct behaviors. They directly and immediately serve values. There is usually no intermediary. Indirect behaviors are more complex. They are intended to influence other people. Chances are, when you use an indirect behavior and it works or doesn't work, you don't know why. As a result, you cannot in any systematic fashion build incrementally and cumulatively a set of powerful behaviors. They involve another human being's perception, values, and behaviors. There are two requirements of indirect behaviors that are not found in direct behaviors. First, when you engage in an indirect behavior, the person you are trying to influence has to interpret your behavior in a certain way, presumably the culturally accepted way. But even if you send out these data fragments and that person interprets them in the culturally appropriate way, they still may not influence the person. He or she is bombarded by signals, data fragments, messages. Your message has to be the most powerful one received at that time.

I can increase the probability that my behavior will get through the filters, will be the dominant information flowing to that person at that time. But there are no guarantees. There is no magic. There is too much variability. What values are you trying to serve when you try to influence people? What are the characteristics of the person you are trying to influence? What is the nature of the organizational relationship between you and that person? Is it the boss, a peer, a subordinate, a client? Built into organizational relationships are all kinds of expectations and aspirations of appropriate and inappropriate behavior. Finally, what is the nature of the interpersonal relationship between you and that person? Is it a stranger, somebody you know, a friend, an enemy, somebody you like, somebody you don't like, somebody you trust, don't trust, somebody who trusts you, somebody who doesn't trust you? There is a large set of issues to be addressed. Our goal, however, is to acquire more and more powerful behaviors incrementally, systematically, and cumulatively.

It is not possible to provide a definitive list of powerful behaviors. There are just too many variables. At best, I can (and will) only give you a few examples of behaviors that work quite well for me and for most people in most situations. But, in addition, I can offer you a set of lenses, a way of looking at situations of potential influence, cooperation, and harmony. These frames will allow you to think through how, if you understand how another person processes information, you might shape the data fragments of your behavior to put the appropriate connections in that person's head. The more you look at the world through those lenses, the more powerful a repertoire of behaviors you will build. Very successful salespersons do exactly that. Every time they make a sale, they debrief themselves to determine what happened, how they got the customer to engage in the behavior they wanted. When they don't get the sale, they analyze what might have been done differently in the situation that would have gotten the behavior they wanted. In this way they continuously build a more powerful repertoire of selling behaviors.

We cannot serve all of our values fully all of the time, of course. Our behaviors require time, energy, knowledge, skill, and other resources. No one has found a single behavior that will simultaneously and fully serve all of our values. We can serve multiple values at a given time, but not all of them fully. So we must choose among them. We must establish priorities. We have to choose which values to attend to at that time and which behaviors to engage in to take care of these values. We make hundreds, maybe thousands, of these choices all day long. For most of us, the choice is essentially automatic. Really semiautomatic, because we are always aware of the context of our behavior. We will engage in certain behaviors in some contexts and not in others. But we engage in the behavior subconsciously. These automatic programs choose the values to serve and then choose the behaviors to engage in. While most of these automatic choices are effective and highly useful to us, there are also many that are ineffective and even dysfunctional. To influence the behavior of others more powerfully, these dysfunctional automatic programs have to be identified and altered.

CHAPTER SEVEN

OVERCOMING OUR OWN AUTOMATION

Our consciousness is fragile, fickle, easily distracted and has a very small capacity, even though in a sense it is where we live and it has an enormous impact on the quality of our lives. We are able to operate with something that small because we have a subconscious. For all practical purposes, it is limitless. All of our automatic processes mentioned in the previous chapter—our skills, beliefs, knowledge, attitudes, and behaviors—are in the subconscious. Programs get into the subconscious in three ways—by being hard-wired (all those infant behaviors, for instance), through learning (say, riding a bike), and through emotional events (experience of the effect of a hot iron on the hand, for example). All of our beliefs, all of our memories, all of our skills, everything we call knowledge, our attitudes, our ongoing emotional responses to stimuli. They are all in the subconscious. We think certain thoughts, feel certain feelings, engage in certain behaviors, all automatically. Most of the stuff of the subconscious is good and useful. But each of us has automatic programs, automatic choices, of values and behaviors that are dysfunctional and counterproductive. Many of them are disastrous with respect to getting cooperation from people. Indeed, we have automatic programs inside of us that stimulate conflict with others. We don't recognize them because the programs have been there for most of our lives, they are automatic, and nearly everyone else has essentially the same programs, so they don't look different and therefore we don't notice them.

To become more powerful in dealing with people, we have to do something about these dysfunctional, automatic programs. We are not going to change the fact that we are on automatic. The issue is the content and quality of those automatic programs when they play.

When a child fails to get something that he or she wants, something that requires the assistance of others, the emotions are predictable. Frustration, anger, disappointment, rejection, disillusionment, rage perhaps. There is a sense of failure.

47

The Shifting Sources of Power and Influence

Children learn early in life that there is a cultural preference for success. They develop a culturally inculcated fear of failure. If it isn't well in place by the time a child gets to kindergarten, the school will take care of it. Schools are very powerful agents for putting fear in children. The cultural necessity of having reasons for things is also instilled early in children's development. They are asked to give reasons for what they do and what they feel. They learn to distinguish parentally acceptable from unacceptable reasons. In short, they learn to lie in order to satisfy parents. Allied with all this, children learn the difference between acceptance and rejection, approval and disapproval, positive and negative self-image. They learn about self-esteem. They learn to want to be accepted and approved and to feel good about themselves. Parents work to teach their child all of these things to aid themselves in influencing their children.

When children fail to get something that they want from others, they have the familiar rush of negative emotions, exacerbated by the knowledge that they have done something socially disapproved; they have failed. They need a reason for the failure and frustration that is acceptable to self-esteem. They don't want to say they're no good or don't deserve what they want. Some children are taught to think that way, and they end up needing psychiatric help; it damages their self-esteem. Coming up with a reason acceptable to self-esteem for failure and frustration is a fairly sophisticated psychological task for a child. But when a culture places a burden upon us, it tends to give us a way to deal with it. Otherwise, we would all be frustrated much of the time. The three-year-old child learns to respond to this challenge by saying, "No fair." This is a child presumably commenting on justice, mercy, ethics, morality, fairness. The child doesn't understand those concepts, but he or she understands that the phrase gives him or her a reason acceptable to self-esteem for what is going wrong. The cause is external. There is a defect in the world that is causing the problem. It is a balm, a salve for the child's burgeoning ego. We learn to say "no fair" at age three and don't stop using it until we die (the final unfairness).

When the child becomes a teenager, the basic message stays the same, only new phrases are added to their repertoire. "You don't understand." "Things are different." "You don't listen to me." "You don't care about me." "You don't love me." "You don't trust me." The teenager is doing exactly what the child was doing. They have to come up with reasons that are acceptable to self-esteem for what is going wrong in their lives, and the most obvious reason is a defect in their parents.

Then, in our early to mid-twenties, parents are no longer plausible reasons because they no longer control and constrain our behavior. Many teenagers believe that once

Overcoming Our Own Automation

they get out from under their parents, life will be idyllic. Then they get out from under their parents and find out life is not idyllic. So employers, spouses, the system, red tape, bureaucracy, city hall, the establishment, all those intractable, intransigent, immoral, insensitive, negative, impossible people we have to deal with, become the new parents. We continue to give excuses, scapegoat, to rationalize. We develop our rationalization program and repeat it everyday in a variety of situations and formats.

If your behavior is important to me, I can try to influence you. I can risk rejection, embarrassment, and failure. Or I can go to a warm, fuzzy, soft, secure, well-supported, place called rationalization. If I try and fail, I can still retreat to rationalization so that I do not have to persist in my attempts to influence you and thereby risk continued failure. That is our default position. Rationalization interferes with interpersonal effectiveness, with our ability to get cooperation. It increases the likelihood that we will end up in dysfunctional conflicts. Because we usually scapegoat the other person—attribute negative characeristics to them to explain our failure to influence them. We have all said, "You can lead a horse to water, but you can't make him drink." That's true, but you can make him exceedingly thirsty before you get him to the water, thereby increasing the probability he will drink. When we gain control over this automatic program and use it less, we increase our effectiveness. We try more often to reach others. We persist. To do this successfully, however, we have to overcome our fear of failure for which this program is a cover, and that is a deeply imbedded automatic program.

There are ways to get automatic programs out of your head, of course, some better than others. Surgery and drugs are used to alter peoples ways of processing information. Brain damage or disease can remove the programming. Electroconvulsive shock therapy has had some, albeit controversial, success. It is important to understand how the brain functions if automatic programs are to be controlled or eliminated, but none of these more intensive techniques are recommended. It would be wonderful to have erase buttons, à la computers, in our brains. We could identify a dysfunctional program, capture it, and just put it in the trash can. That's not the way our brains work. There is no erase program. But you can learn in a relatively short time painless approaches to overriding the automatic program. You can go into your brain and alter what we might simply call a stimulus-response relationship. You probably learned to drive a car in the United States. If you have subsequently driven a car in a foreign country with different rules for the side on which you drive, you know that an adjustment is required. You have an automatic program that is totally functional in a given environment. You take it into another environment, and it's a disaster.

The Shifting Sources of Power and Influence

Twenty years ago, I conducted my first seminar in London. I flew in overnight on a Friday to get there early Saturday morning. I wanted the weekend to adjust to the time change. I hired a car, but I wasn't naive. I knew those people drive on the other side of the road. I was prepared (or so I thought), but I was a little tired. There was very light traffic when I started from the airport. Everything was fine until I got to the first traffic circle ("roundabout"). My automatic program told me to go right, counterclockwise, which I did. I was immediately confronted by a huge truck. Fortunately for me, the driver of the truck was English and knew he was near Heathrow. He was on the look-out for Yanks. So I survived what thereafter became for me a significant emotional event.

For the next few days, I consciously overrode my automatic program for driving. My consciousness had to be continuously brought back to the task of driving a new way. Fortunately, there were cues for bringing my easily distracted consciousness back to the task. One was other cars. Part of my problem on Saturday morning was there weren't any cars around. There wasn't anything to alert me to go the correct way. For the remainder of the trip, other cars were a constant reminder. Every time I wanted to make a right-hand turn, I was hoping that the car in front of me would make it first to remind me I could copy it. I also had signs. At home, I can process signs automatically. Every time there was a sign in England, I rehearsed what I was going to do at the next intersection. Finally, the car itself reinforced the new rules. The location of the drivers seat, the steering wheel, the gear shift, the rear view mirror—all conformed with driving on the left side of the road. If you want a real thrill, rent an American car in England. It is much more difficult to drive the new way when the environment is reinforcing the old way.

What I learned, because I wanted to drive a car over there, was a general method for overriding an automatic program that was dysfunctional. It was not easy. Everything in the environment was new, distracting. Everything tended to pull the consciousness away from driving, but I couldn't allow my consciousness to be diverted for even a second. If there was an emergency during that second, I would revert to the old automatic program, which has a neurological advantage, until I had enough conscious rehearsals for the new program.

Let me give you another example of overriding automatic programs, this one involving value/behavior relationships. Humans seek comfort and the absence of pain or discomfort. Touch the hand or foot of an infant with a sharp object, and it automatically pulls away. There are people who have reprogrammed their brains so that they no longer automatically move away from painful stimuli. If you go into a gym, you will see a sign on the wall. "No pain, no gain." All those people in the gym are joyfully, voluntarily, undergoing pain. Pain that feels good because they perceive that the pain is a sign that they are making progress with respect to a valued outcome. They have made a new neurological linkage in their brains between pain and their values. They have overridden the automatic response to pain.

There are three conditions necessary for successfully overriding an automatic program. First, we have to identify the program and our use of it as automatic. Second, we must have an alternative program. Finally, we have to install the new program using a quite specific method. That's not what we have been taught. We have been taught that once we discover a dysfunctional or counterproductive program in our brains, we should be able to overcome it by will power, by self-control, by discipline. Those approaches don't work very well for most people. Every time we say we are not going to think, feel, or do something, we increase the likelihood we will do exactly what we say we do not want to do because of the structure of the brain.

We walk into a restaurant and look at the dessert tray. We've have been eating too many desserts. Chocolate mousse is our favorite, but we are not going to have it for dessert tonight. While we are saying that, we're salivating. Our brain is rehearsing the wonderful experience of eating chocolate mousse. We then order a salad with our entrée so we can rationalize the chocolate mousse for dessert. This is called the Wallenda effect. When the Great Wallenda fell to his death, it wasn't a dangerous walk. The tightrope wasn't particularly high, the equipment was fine, he seemed to be in great health, the weather wasn't bad. Yet he fell to his death. The difference was (as reported by his widow) that, for the first time in his career, all he could think about before the walk was not falling. In his subconscious, every time he was telling himself not to fall, he was falling. He was rehearsing falling.

So we need an alternative program, not the absence of a current automatic program, and then we have to install it in our subconsciousness through repetition. Here is the one I use: "Never expect anyone to engage in behavior that serves your values unless you give that person adequate reason to do so." Adequate reason doesn't necessarily mean arguments and evidence. It may be an emotional appeal; it may be an indirect appeal. If you are not doing what I want you to do, or if you are doing something I don't want you to do, I have only one explanation. I have not yet, by my behavior, given you adequate reason to do anything else. Your current pattern of behavior makes sense to you. Under what conditions are you going to change your behavior? When I, by my behavior, change the sense you presently have in your head about your current pattern of behavior. Sometimes, we try to influence people with phrases such as "It's your job," "It's what you're paid to do," "It's your responsibility," and "It's our expectation." These aren't adequate reasons for most people. The alternative program drives me away from rationalization. It drives me toward taking responsibility for my effectiveness. Above all, it moves me toward action.

But just knowing an alternative program isn't enough. To overcome the power of the subconscious automatic program of rationalization, the new program has to be rehearsed repeatedly. If you want the new program to be a permanent part of your subconscious, you have to repeat it to yourself, under two very specific conditions, 12-15 times a day for 14 or more days (i.e., about two hundred repetitions).

You can understand the statement as soon as you read it. You can memorize the statement in 15 seconds, but that's not installation. If that were installation, we would all be what we want to be. The new program has to have enough neurological practice to be powerful enough to override the old program. Put it on a card on your desk. Tie it to some automatic behavior, such as brushing your teeth. Use a physical reminder, at least at first. Put your ring on the other hand, a ribbon on a finger. Or put a copy of the statement on the refrigerator, on the mirror, in the drawer, in your car, on your desk, on your telephone, in your wallet.

You'll still have to change the location every few days, because it will soon become transparent to the consciousness. The brain is, among other things, an exception-reporting device. When you walk into a room, the visual information from the room hits your eye, bypasses your consciousness, and goes directly to your subconsciousness. It compares what is reported with the image that is in your memory bank. If the comparison is fine, your brain doesn't disturb you. If something is moved or missing, it is reported to your consciousness. The system is not infallible, but, in general, it works well, except when you are trying to install an override program. Then the brain's predilection to report only new information works against installing the new program into your subconscious.

Identification and repetition are still not enough. Even if the new program is in your head for the rest of your life, it would be totally useless to you unless, in the repetitions, you have tied it neurologically to the appropriate stimulus. This means you have to be honest with yourself. You have to determine some stimulus that triggers the rationalization response. A person, a topic, a situation that you know you rationalize about. Then, every time you rehearse the new program, you picture that stimulus and you see and hear yourself responding with the new program. You are now neurologically, through the powers of your imagination, creating a new stimulus-response program in your brain. You vividly see the stimulus and see and hear yourself responding with the statement. Eventually, when the stimulus occurs in a real situation, it goes to the new neurological destination that you have prepared by rehearsal.

If you want this technique to work powerfully and quickly, you will add one more dimension. It is not essential, but it is easy to learn and beneficial and improves the power of this method. We now know that if you are in a certain brain state when you want to learn something new, you will learn it much more quickly. Herbert Benson, MD, of Harvard University brought into the laboratory a number of people who were using Transcendental Meditation and tested them. He discovered that not only did their respiration, heart beat, and blood pressure decrease, but they also altered their brain states when they moved into meditation. If you trigger this relaxation response before you do the rehearsals, they tend to be absorbed much more quickly. You are also going to get hooked on the relaxation, which allows you to trigger the response several times a day, thereby decreasing the unnecessary energy you and I have been taught to put out every day through ongoing muscle tension. You can also use the "relaxation response" to trigger a calmer emotional response when you go into situations that might otherwise trigger dysfunctional anxiety or tension. There is some speculation that the relaxation response may be one of the reasons we were veritable learning machines between birth and age three. The speculation is that it is the natural state of infants when they are awake and greatly facilitates learning.

There are two popular generic approaches to the relaxation technique on instructional audiotapes. One is called "Autogenic" and the other "Progressive." They are each about 25 minutes long. Used once a day for about two weeks, the tape should instill the relaxation response. With the progressive tape, you clench your fists tighter and tighter, hold at maximum tightness, and then relax them. It takes you through all of the muscle groups. It is an adaptation of yoga exercises. Your brain begins to understand how to do this more quickly and efficiently. At the end of two weeks of practice, you should be able to just say relax and the brain will send signals to the various muscle groups. The process also changes the brain's state and makes it more susceptible to new programming. The autogenic tape is similar, except that it uses the brain as an imaginative device and asks you to think of some muscle as heavy or warm. This process relaxes that muscle group. Again, you are just rehearsing learning through repetition. Some versions of the tapes will paint an idyllic scene, such as a beach or a mountain, to assist in the relaxation response.

With these techniques, you don't have to find every stimulus that triggers rationalization in you. If you use it for one stimulus that triggers the rationalization response, there will be a ripple affect. Your subconscious begins to send other stimuli to the new response. The old automatic programs are still in your brain, however. If you become exhausted, highly emotional, or under the influence of alcohol or other drugs and the old stimulus occurs, the brain may very well go to the old response. You can't do anything about that, except try not to be in those situations. The more you rehearse, the less likely a reversion is, but the old program is always there and may play from time to time.

A curious phenomenon may occur in the middle of your rehearsals. A stimulus may arrive and the brain will not know where to send it. The two neurological responses in your brain, the old rationalization response and the new rational response, are equal in strength. The stimulus bounces back and forth between the two. While this is a strange sensation, it should be encouraging to you. This tells you that after a few more rehearsals, you will be over the threshold. You also begin to understand that you are creating, in the present rehearsals, a series of new responses to future situations. When the future situations occur, you automatically respond the new way, but you are consciously aware you formerly responded the old way, with rationalization. You feel like a spectator of your own emotions or thoughts of behavior. You are, in a way, a puppet, but you are also the puppeteer. Until now, the old automatic programs, put in your head by other people without your permission, before you had any critical faculty, were done by the puppeteer.

Overcoming rationalization isn't the only application of these techniques. It can also be used to overcome tension, anxiety, distress, guilt, blame, hatred, anger, jealousy, and all fears. Take the latter emotion and behavior. You are born fearless. There are no primordial fears. You can startle an infant, but infants have no built-in fear. You have to learn fear. Studies indicate that the infant's learned fear has a great deal to do with the facial expressions of its mother. She subconsciously sends just barely perceptible cues that the infant picks up. There is no innate fear of falling, no innate fear of heights. The child very early in its life picks up fear cues from the mother. You can put a snake in a baby's crib, and it's not going to be afraid. It is just another object in its environment, a resource to be played with. But the first time the child does encounter a snake or some other adult-frightening object, the reactions from the adults present introduce it to fear. We have built an elaborate rationalization around fear. "It keeps us safe," we say. It may, in some ways, keep us safe, but it is also unnecessary, uncomfortable, and unreliable. It can lead to panic or paralysis. But most of us acquire fears in our childhoods, and then pass them along to the next generation.

It is dysfunctional, counterproductive, and plain stupid to give someone a fear response if something is, in fact, dangerous and common in their environment. If something is common and dangerous, you wouldn't think of making your children afraid of it. You would give them knowledge and skill so they know how to deal with it, thereby reducing the likelihood that they will be injured. Children born and raised in an environment with poisonous snakes are given knowledge and skill—not fear. Children born and raised in an environment with dangerous cars are given knowledge and skill—not fear. We are given fear of failure. We are given fear of rats and snakes, and bats, and spiders. We are given fear of embarrassment, we are given fear of loss of job. We are given fear of death and dying. And those fears have a lot to do with our patterns of behavior. All of them are dysfunctional.

If you were able to reduce your tendency to rationalize, you would be more powerful. You would try more often. You wouldn't be as afraid, and you could develop effective, automatic responses. Of course, there is a price to be paid for all of this. You shut forever a trapdoor we have all had since age three. There is great fear in doing this because of our socialization. If you take this step, for the rest of your life you will have to take full responsibility for everything you think, everything you feel, every behavior you engage in. You won't be able to say that "he makes me angry," or "she drives me up a wall," or "that makes my blood boil." Each of these statements is emotional suicide. Every time you talk that way, you are rehearsing failure, giving control of your emotions to other people and to events. You are doing negative rehearsal. "He makes me angry." Every time I say that what am I doing? I am increasing the likelihood I will feel anger the next time I see him. "She drives me up a wall." Every time I say that to myself or someone else, I increase the likelihood I will feel driven up a wall when I encounter her. Why would we do something that stupid? Why would we hand control of our emotions over to external stimuli? To avoid responsibility for what we don't want to feel inside. It's too high a price to pay!

CHAPTER EIGHT

INFLUENCING THEM TO DO WHAT YOU WANT THEM TO DO

Now that you have overcome your fear of failure, decreased your tendency to rationalize, increased your tendency to take action, and taken responsibility for your effectiveness, how are you going to build a repertoire of more effective behaviors? How are you going to increase your power? Let me start with figure 1, page 58, the world's most accurate organizational chart. It varies significantly from organizational charts that you have been accustomed to. You and your values occupy the center. This starting point is not pessimistic or cynical. Both the cynic and I believe everyone acts out of something inside themselves. The cynic believes that the things that are inside people are fundamentally and necessarily narrow and self-centered. I don't. We all work out of some preexisting states inside of our heads, a portion of which I call our values. I am not suggesting that there is not a sense of ethics, morality, goodness, principle, justice, and altruism in people. I am suggesting that they are either in someone's value system or they aren't. And you are not likely to put them there if they aren't.

If the person you want to influence has these characteristics, appeal to them. If they don't, appeal to something that is in them, because, in any case, they are going to engage in behaviors designed by them to serve their values. We start from this core of our values and engage in behaviors. We make phone calls, answer phone calls, write memos, read memos, go to meetings, call meetings, have informal conversations with people, write reports. We engage in behaviors that involve other people—bosses, patients, peers, suppliers, subordinates, government, media, board members. You can draw your own chart. Most of the time when we are engaged in behavior involving these other people, we are trying to change, to influence, their behavior. If they respond as we want, we expect that our values will be served. The people we want to influence have multiple behaviors available to them. Anybody we are trying to influence is being subjected to influence from many other people who don't necessarily want the behavior that we want. Our behavior must get through the other person's filters. It has to be stronger than the other messages trying to get

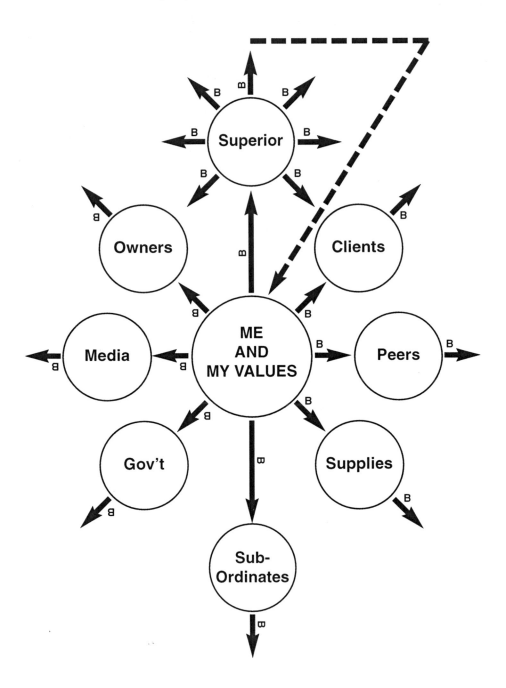

FIGURE 1—World's most accurate organizational chart.

through. And when it gets through, it has to indicate which behavior the person should enact to best serve his or her values.

That last statement is extraordinarily important. Our behavior needs to be designed very carefully and consciously so that the other person comes to perceive that the behavior we want is the best thing he or she can do to take care of what is important to him or her. We must look to the person's interests, values, and perception of how he or she processes information. I'll use myself as an example. At a recent conference at which I was a faculty presenter for one day, I arrived at the hotel late the night before. I didn't want to have to check out at noon (the regular check out time) on the meeting day. I wanted to have lunch and relax a little, not rush back to my room and pack my bag at the lunch break. The morning of the seminar I stopped at the desk and asked if there was any possibility of a late checkout. I told the clerk I was conducting a seminar for seventy-five people that day. I was told that the manager had said that there couldn't be any exceptions whatsoever that day. They had a full house and couldn't accommodate any late checkouts. I thanked the clerk and went back to my room. I called the conference organizer and asked him if he would be good enough to call the hotel catering and sales people and see if my checkout time could be extended. A few minutes later, I received a call telling me that I had until 3 p.m. to check out. This is an example of indirect influence. It also illustrates what one sometimes needs to do to get the desired outcome. Do you see the reasons the second approach worked while the first did not?

While this is a modest example, it points to much larger possibilities. Nearly anything is possible. All resources are available and under the control of people. But the direct approach may not be best. An indirect approach to influence, such as that used in the scenario above, may be more effective. Rather than my calling the manager, it was much better for the person who had brought 150 people (the total number in the program) to the hotel for a week to make a call to the hotel people responsible for the event—sales people, catering people. They, of course, wanted to please the client, and so they called the manager (with whom they had much more influence than I), and I got the result I wanted.

There is a process to influencing others and some rules that make the process effective. The first rule is, whenever you are trying to influence anyone, get very clear in your head what behavior or performance, what observable, measurable, quantifiable outcome you want from that person or group. What behavioral change do you want from the person, or what outcome of behavior, what performance? Eventually, that behavior or performance is going to have to be in that person's head. Sometimes, people don't do what we want them to do because they don't know what we want. We have not been specific and concrete enough. Fuzzy notions of what we want from other people won't do. Make it measurable, observable, quantifiable.

The second thing that you need clearly in your head is an understanding of the other person's values. The other person has values that he or she wants to have satisfied. You must add that element to your equation. You have to have what you want from them and what they want from the world clearly in mind. People often stop at this point, thinking that they have no idea what the other person's values are. You would be surprised how much knowledge you have about people's values. You have been influencing people all your life, and you know a great deal about what is important to them.

Let me give you an example that I hope is persuasive. Suppose you go to a bank to make a transaction. You get into the now familiar single queue. As you move up in the line, you notice there are four tellers behind the counter, and one of them is in a bad mood. This teller is, by your interpretation of the data fragments of his behavior, rude, surly and uncooperative, being difficult with each customer who comes up to the counter. As you move farther up the line, you observe instances of unusual politeness at the front of the line. The person at the front of the line who notices he is about to get the surly teller offers to let the person behind him go ahead of him. But that person has no desire to encounter the surly teller and declines the offer. Then you get to the head of the line and discover that you will be served by the surly teller. If you want to have a very high probability of getting pleasant, efficient behavior from the person, if you want to get that person to treat you unlike he has treated any other person in line, in what behavior should you engage? You know the answer. You should smile. Have a relaxed, open body posture. Give a pleasant greeting. Say hello. Make eye contact. Call him by name. (The teller has a name badge, but no one ever calls him by name.) Compliment him. Empathize with him. "I guess ever since they put in these 24-hour teller machines, you must get a lot of hassles in this bank." You would probably be the first customer to empathize with him about the threat to his job that those automatic tellers pose.

What values in the teller are you touching when you engage in those behaviors? Esteem, respect, acceptance! You are giving him a sample of the value satisfaction available from you. That behavior is very likely to alter his affective states, given the contrast of your behavior toward him and that of the previous people in the line. That teller will likely respond positively to your behavior, because he will want it to continue and he understands that his behavior is key to that continuation. He perceives that he is getting a flow of value satisfaction from you and will understand that it will continue if he gives you a flow of value satisfaction back in the way of cordiality and efficiency. In short, you and everyone else knows what to do to get the behavior we want from the teller. Is that therefore what we do? No! We tend to do exactly the opposite.

The people before you in line did not engage in behaviors that had any probability whatsoever of getting both the affect and the behavior that they wanted from the teller. They approached him in a surly, aggressive manner. Cold, no eye contact, stiff, tense, no smile, no greeting. "I would like to make this transaction, please." The teller's understandable perception would be, "I have had a bunch of lousy people today." No one knows if the behavior problem started with the teller or with an early client. All we know is there is an unfortunate choreography going on. People walk up nasty, get a nasty response, and have no notion at all that their nastiness, their surliness, their coolness reinforces precisely the behavior they don't want from the teller. What is the reason that most of us do the exact opposite of what we should (and know how to) do to get the response we want? Fear. Fear of failure, fear of rejection, fear of embarrassment. "What if I walk up to the teller full of cordiality and friendliness, and he says, 'What's it to you? What do you want?' What if I my good intentions are rejected?"

When we were children, we learned to trade a 95 percent success rate to protect against a five percent failure rate. When you were a child, you were willing to do all kinds of things you're not willing to do as an adult. For example, you were sitting outside of your house one day eating your favorite ice cream cone. You're five years old and a six-year-old neighbor comes down the street. You're a nice person and you're feeling generous, so you offer him a taste of your ice cream cone. But he just got dumped on by his parents and he is full of bitterness and frustration. He's looking for a dumpee, and you're perfect. So he says, "I don't want any of your crummy ice cream cone." Unfortunately, what you learned that day was never to do that again. Never make myself vulnerable. Never extend yourself. Never take a chance, especially if the other person seems to be in a bad mood.

It costs to be effective; it involves risks. You have to open yourself up to possible rejection. Sometimes you get burned, but the 95 percent success rate is well worth the five percent failure rate. Unfortunately, we have been taught not to risk it, not to do what is likely to work. All of these defense mechanisms, all of these rationalizations, roar up inside of us.

So each of us knows a good deal about other people's values, both because we have appealed to them throughout our lives and because we, likewise, have many of them. People want security, autonomy, appreciation and gratitude, recognition and acceptance, approval, success, achievement. They want fun, excitement, challenge. But the number one item on that list is self-esteem. How we feel about ourselves. How do you think Marines get 18-year-olds to throw their bodies on grenades. To crawl through mine fields. Those feats are the price of admission into the Marines. If being a Marine makes you feel terrific about yourself, those feats are the cost of self-esteem. It's a high cost but it's worth it in their minds. While we may not go to the same lengths to satisfy our need for self-esteem, all of us have it, to some significant degree, as a primary value.

We can also identify the values of others by watching their behavior and talking to them and by asking people who know them better than we do. If you engage in conversation with people and listen, they will reveal what is important to them. You may have to filter the information, of course, because one strategy for maintaining our self-esteem is to lie to ourselves (and others) about what our values are. But you can discover much about another person's value system, certainly enough to be effective with them. But the task does not end there.

While many people buy into the notion that values drive behavior, they make too simple an assumption. They assume that if people have certain values, they will, thereby, engage in certain behaviors. As a corollary, if people engage in certain behaviors, we can pretty much understand their values. Not quite. It's not a one-to-one relationship. That assumption causes us to make three errors. If you get the notion in your head that values drive behavior directly, you might try to surround yourself with people who have the appropriate values. That's not a particularly useful approach. It may be awkward to tell your boss that you've been watching his or her behaviors, that you have noticed some value gaps in them, and that you feel they are beyond remediation and that he/she ought to resign. Such behavior on your part is unlikely to serve your values. Your resignation is about the only likely outcome in such a scenario. And about the only place that we can use this strategy is when we are hiring subordinates.

But in all job interviews, even if the candidate doesn't want the job, the candidate is apt to engage in behaviors that lead us to believe he or she has values that he or she doesn't have. Should we hire that person, we usually discover the error of our decision one day after the probationary period. I'm not saying we shouldn't interview people. I am saying that even if we do accurately assess their values, this may very well not predict subsequent patterns of behavior. And that is what we are ultimately after. So the interview, whether for a job or for any purpose, is a weak way, a very limited way, of ensuring that people will do what we want them to do.

Influencing Them To Do What You Want Them To Do

A second error is to assume that the other person's values can be changed. This goes back to my discussion of so-called "organizational culture." Our flawed reasoning is that if we change the values of the people around us, the likelihood that they will engage in desired behaviors will be increased. I don't know how to change people's values. Are we going to provide significant emotional events for the people around us? Are we going to send out a few data fragments and their brains are going to melt into this new value system that we have composed for them? I don't think so. Even if we did change somebody's values, we are unlikely to get the behavior that we want. And even if we could change people's values, somebody else would come along and change them back.

The third, and most common, error we make is believing that if we serve someone's values, he or she will engage in behavior that serves ours. In the early 1950s, Abraham Maslow first published his needs hierarchy. He called them needs; I'll call them values. He established a fundamental set of human values and placed them in a hierarchical pyramid. He said that once a given level of needs is served, the next group becomes active, and so on. Several years later, he recanted on the strict pyramid-like structure of the hierarchy, but by then the pyramid had become popular and his self-criticism was largely ignored. It is still published in its original form, despite Maslow's discovery that it is not as hierarchical as he originally thought. But what people in organizations did and are still doing is to seize and misapply the hierarchy as something magical. Now they felt that they knew what is important to people. Now they knew what people's values are. The manager gives value satisfaction to employees in the belief that they will then engage in more of the behaviors the manager wants from them.

It doesn't work that way. But they put carpets on the floor, paint the walls a soft green, put rubber plants in corners, hang pictures on the walls, pipe in Muzak®, and wait for the people to take off in performance. At best, they are likely to get a behavioral blip, what is called the Hawthorne Effect. It doesn't sustain over time. So some managers assume they didn't go high enough in Maslow's Needs Hierarchy. Now they offered social and affiliative needs/value satisfactions. The organization is to be one big happy family. We are talking picnics, parties, ball teams, clubs. It still doesn't work. But they persist. They assume they still hadn't gone high enough in the hierarchy, so they go to the top—self-actualization. They provide growth, development, challenge, self-actualization, thinking that employees would, in return, give them the behavior they sought. They fail again.

Giving people value satisfaction is, by no means, an effective way to influence their subsequent behavior. Sometimes they will reciprocate. Often they will not. Yet, we attempt it all the time, with spouses, children, friends, colleagues, staff, superiors, etc. And then we wonder why it doesn't work. We are hurt, are let down, feel betrayed. "I treat them well. The least they can do is give me some of what I want in return." You misunderstand the basic principles of human influence. Giving in order to get is not a very powerful technique for reasons we will discover below. Note: In the bank example we gave a *sample* of available value satisfaction to elicit the desired response.

One way to understand the weakness of reciprocity is to ask the question, "Does money motivate?" Most people will say "Yes" or "To a certain extent" or "If there is enough money offered" or "For some people." Some will say "No. It is a satisfier not a motivator." All of these answers are wrong, based on a misunderstanding of human behavior and influence. The question is nonsensical. It literally makes no sense. Does Tuesday motivate? How about purple? A glass of water? Those are equally sensible, or nonsensible questions. Let me ask a different question. Do most people, however differentially, place some instrumental value on money? The answer is "yes." Whether money motivates, however, depends not only on how much people value money and how much money is offered, but also, and most critically, on the perceived relationship of the money to the desired behavior. Anything that an individual values, intrinsically or instrumentally, is a **potential** source of motivation. Whether it in fact motivates depends upon the perceived relationship between it and the behavior or performance sought by the influencer.

The issue, again, is one of perception, of a personal, fragile, subjective, idiosyncratic, arbitrary, infinitely malleable state in someone's head. Do you have any hourly employees in your organization? What, in fact, are the minimum conditions necessary for an hourly employee to have access to an hour's wage? Most people respond that "it is to be there for an hour." Not true! It is to be perceived to have been there for an hour, to be on the payroll and have an hour go by. Do you have an idea of how creatively people can meet those conditions, collect their wages, and give you none of the behavior you want? You probably have better examples than I do. Most people in this country are paid in a way that has little effect on the patterns of their behavior. They are paid wages and salaries, fringe benefits, and working conditions. But those things don't motivate. They attract a pool of people ready to come and take them and, if those people perceive they are getting more of these things than they might get elsewhere, turnover will be reduced. But it doesn't buy day-to-day behavior, because a strong perceived relationship between behavior or performance on the one hand and receipt of the money on the other has not been established. Until the two are connected, contingently, inside somebody's perception, one does not influence the other.

Influencing Them To Do What You Want Them To Do

We pour value satisfaction—wages, salaries, fringe benefits, working conditions—all over employees and then expect some behavior in return. Why should they give it to us? Because it's the right thing to do? If we give them a Protestant work ethic sermonette, will that change their behavior? Maybe they will do it out of gratitude. After all we are serving their values. Won't they want to serve ours in return? Not necessarily. Gratitude is one of the shallowest and shortest lived of human emotions. The last time I checked the research literature, eternal gratitude was lasting about 3.2 days. Of course, even when we don't get what we want, we foolishly continue to pour value satisfaction on them. We continue the wages, salaries, fringe benefits, and working conditions of marginal people. We even continue to provide wages and fringes to people who are a net drag on the resources of the organization, because it costs us too much, individually and personally, to get rid of them. For years, managers have pleaded that, if only people were paid more money, the managers could get the behavior they want. It doesn't work. You can pay them more and still not alter their behavior one bit. If you want to use money to influence behavior, and I am not suggesting that you do, how do you have to structure it for people? How do you connect it in their perception with the behavior you want? What are the systems for doing that? Piece rate, commissions, performance contracting, pay for performance, fee for service (the physician's form of piece rate), and bonuses if tied to behavior or performance. That's what managers and executives all too frequently fail to do. I am not necessarily suggesting that you attempt to change the compensation system in your organization even if you could. That requires some subtleties not covered in this discussion. I am simply trying to provide an extended example, by using money, of the basic principle of human influence. If you can connect the two concepts inside people's heads, the behavior you want from them and the value satisfaction they want, you can get anybody to do anything you want.

An illustration from the Bible may be useful here. We are told in the Old Testament that Abraham was willing to engage in a most unusual (one might say heinous) behavior toward his most beloved and innocent son, Issac. He was willing to sacrifice him. To cut his throat, decapitate him, and burn his body on an altar. Why? Because he perceived that God had commanded him to do so and doing God's will was the prime value in his life. His behavior, just like everyone else's, is a function of his values mediated by his perception of the relationship of that behavior to his values.

To use our behavior more effectively this way, we must be willing to accept certain costs and risks. Earlier, I discussed the difference between behaviors that directly and immediately result in value satisfaction without the need to influence anyone (which I will now label A behaviors) and those behaviors that serve our values

TRADE-OFFS

CHOICES

CONFLICTS

PRIORITIES

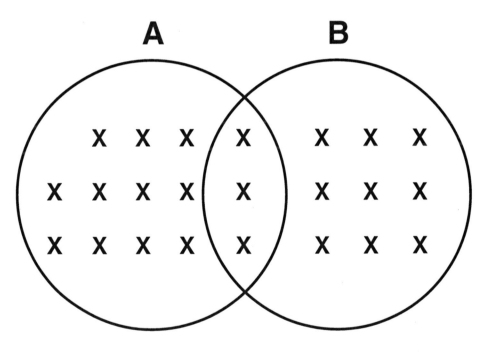

FIGURE 2—A and B Behaviors

Influencing Them To Do What You Want Them To Do

because they influence others (which I will now label B behaviors). In figure 2, page 66, A and B behaviors are displayed in a different configuration to make a different point. A behaviors, I call them feel-good behaviors, are available to us all day long. Eat a good meal, watch a good ball game. Watch a good TV show, a concert, a ballet, an opera. There are all sorts of ways we can use our time, energy, and other personal resources to serve our values. We engage other people with no intent to influence their behavior. but rather to derive a value satisfaction from our behavior toward them. We simply do a kindness for a friend, or vent our frustrations on a child, or meet an obligation to a parent. The behavior, in a sense, bounces off that person and comes immediately back to us in the form of a value satisfaction. It may, for example, enhance our self-esteem. There are numerous A behaviors that feel good even though they may in some cases involve other human beings. But they are not what the influence game is all about.

Influence is a matter of B behaviors. It is about behaviors that serve our values because they influence other people's behavior. Notice the slight overlapping in the relationship. Unfortunately, for most of us, there aren't too many behaviors that both feel good and are effective. We would love to believe that effective behaviors feel good, but very often the truth is they have costs and risks associated with them. If you want to be more powerful, you will have to use more B behaviors and give up some A behaviors. Our biological bias favors A behaviors over B behaviors, so we engage in A behaviors, hoping they will be effective. When they are not, we blame the other person. That's not what power is all about. Power is about our willingness to use the B behaviors. I indicated above that I am unable to give a definitive list of B behaviors because of the complexity of interpersonal relationships. But I did promise some examples of what, for most people, will prove to be powerful approaches to influence.

One of the most powerful behaviors ever invented for influencing the behavior of others is a request for help. If you're asked to help someone, you feel good, valuable, worthwhile. It gives you power in the relationship. It makes the requester vulnerable to you because you can turn the person down. At least implicitly, it gives you some ownership of the task. You are entitled to some of the recognition upon completion of the task. The requester has said that you are the kind of person who helps people. When you respond with the requested help, you get a rush of positive emotions, plus a huge fringe benefit. The person owes you. You can feel altruistic and put money in the bank at the same time. If all these things about the request for help are true, why don't we use it more? Because people don't want to give power to others. They don't want to be vulnerable or share ownership. They don't want to share recognition or be indebted. We won't do what works, because we won't pay the price. If you want more power, ask more people for help. Yes, sometimes they will cash in more chits than you thought you gave them, but that's the risk you take.

If I truly want your help with some problem I am having, I should say, "I have a problem and I need your help." But that is costly and risky, so I choose a phrase that is safe and easy but not very powerful, "We have a problem." If it works, I have not been vulnerable and I owe you nothing, because it is "our" problem we are working on. If you don't give me what I want (which is likely), I can walk away calling you names and mumbling that "you are not a team player. You doesn't believe in the mission of this organization. You're only out for yourself." This is not very effective but it is safe and easy.

An even more powerful move is to give people recognition. When you give recognition, it goes right to the bottom line of self-esteem, but only in exchange for the behavior or performance you want the person to repeat in the future. People get so little recognition in their lives, except when things go wrong. Then there is plenty of negative recognition. When I go as a consultant to an organization, I inevitably hear, "When we do it right, we hear nothing. When we do it wrong, we hear everything." Criticism seems far more common than praise in our organizational life. And yet there is no known satiation point for human recognition. In all of recorded history, no one has been heard to say, "I've had it up to here. If anybody else tells me again how good I am, I'll quit." Is that a problem in your organization? At exit interviews, do people say they are so overburdened with recognition that they have to seek abuse just to balance their lives? I doubt it.

You can break this negative pattern. Maybe, once a week, for 15 minutes, perhaps on a Friday afternoon, dash off two or three brief notes of recognition, praise, appreciation, of thanks to people who have engaged in behavior you want to see repeated. Watch your power grow. Write it in your own handwriting so that it doesn't look as though it is boilerplate off of a word processor. They will be eager to repeat the behavior, as will those who see how it is rewarded. It may be the only such note they have ever received or will ever receive. It's physical. It's tangible. It shows you are sincere. They can show it to others. Some of them will carry it in their wallets for the rest of their lives. They will take it out and read it again and again whenever they need a lift. If your response is that you don't have time for writing such letters, then you don't have time for power.

Why don't we do more of it? Because of the costs and risks we perceive we will have to bear in using it. Managers are concerned that, "If I give you recognition, you will think you are better than you are. You will want more money. You will want a promotion." "If I give you recognition, people will think you are responsible for the success of my department." "I don't get any recognition; why should you." "If you give too much recognition, you cheapen the currency." We have a thousand reasons for not being effective. Sure, there are costs and risks for giving recognition. We want to be powerful, but we don't want to pay the freight.

As you already know, the easiest way to get the boss to enthusiastically endorse and help implement one of your ideas is to give ownership of the idea. But bosses often resist ownership of ideas until they know they are going to work. I have an intermediate strategy for you. Make it absolutely clear to the boss that, if the idea does work, the boss gets all the credit and, if it fails, you get all the blame. It is going to happen that way anyway. There is nothing magnanimous about offering the inevitable. Your current attitude is probably that if it's your idea and it's good for the organization, the boss should endorse and implement it and you should get credit for it. You want too much. If you need resources from the boss, they will be provided only because he or she perceives that doing so is the best thing to be done in the service of the boss's values. Abide by this principle and, once again, watch your power grow.

You can also enjoy a surge in your power if you begin to take total responsibility for all communications in which you are involved. Ordinarily, when there is a breakdown in communication between us and others, we presume, using one of our automatic programs, that the other person has misunderstood or misinterpreted our message. We will either say this or show it in our body language. "No, that's not what I meant. No, you misunderstood. You are not paying attention." We put the burden, the responsibility for the breakdown in communication, on others, whose filters will then shut down immediately. You can gain power by accepting responsibility for the breakdown saying things such as, "I don't think I said that very well." "I don't think I made that very clear." "Let me try that again." The other person now won't feel threatened, will know that you're not going to put a burden on him or her, and will listen with filters wide open. Now you can influence the person. The same is true when you are the recipient of someone else's attempt at communication. When there is a breakdown, when you don't understand, don't say, "That was very confusing" or "That wasn't very clear." Instead say, "It is really important to me that I understand you and I am not certain that I do. Please help me." These phrases do not trip off the tongue easily, but they are, nonetheless, powerful. Practice them and watch how much more effective you become with others.

Each of these B behaviors, and myriad others, if used repeatedly, can be very powerful. They go against our automatic programming and involve some risk, but they are key ingredients of influence. Using B behaviors is not, however, enough. While you have to take on more B behaviors, you must also give up some A behaviors. Each of us engages in behaviors that produce conflict with other people. You may not even know you are doing it. Do you look for deference from people below you in the organization? Do you give unnecessary commands? Do you interrupt subordinates and not allow them to interrupt back? We all display these counterproductive behaviors, and they cause dysfunctional conflict for us.

A common scenario will illustrate the point. A client is coming to see you at 10 o'clock Tuesday morning. At 10 o'clock, your secretary tells you he has arrived. The secretary is waiting for you to engage in some type of behavior, to know what to do with Mr. Jones. Let's say that you're anxious to see the client, so you say, "Show him in." That is a double command. You are commanding the secretary to command the client to come in. This is your turf. This is your threshold. You, not the secretary and not the client, give commands. You are reestablishing the asymmetry of your relationship with the secretary. You can use commands with her. She is not to use them with you. If you don't think that is what is going on, answer this question: When was the last time your secretary said, "No, you get out here." Sounds ludicrous, doesn't it? Let me reinforce this point in another way. What would trip off your tongue, without any conscious processing whatsoever, if, instead of the client, the visitor were the chairman of your organization's board. I suspect you might say something like, "I'll be right out." No threshold. No command. No ego trip this time.

We engage in such feel-good behavior routinely, and it interferes with our effectiveness. We seek deference. We seek dominance. We interrupt. We give commands. We aren't egomaniacs, but the behaviors feel good. Nowhere is all this behavior more pronounced than in organizational staff meetings. Almost universally, there is a belief that there are too many of them and they are too long and not productive enough. Meetings tend to be jammed with feel-good behaviors that interfere with effectiveness and create conflicts. The signs are unmistakable. Pontificating, posturing, monologues in the presence of captive audiences, soliloquies, king of the hill, lord of the manor, Arthur and his court, the crystal through whom all messages must pass. Surely, you have seen such behaviors at meetings. Have you also noticed that the meetings you chair are qualitatively superior to the ones you simply attend? As chairs, we engage in precisely the same behaviors that alienate us when we go to other people's meetings. We don't notice because we're having such a good time.

So, if you want to be more effective and more powerful, you must overcome your tendency to rationalize and your fear of failure, take 100 percent responsibility for all of your communications, give up feel-good behaviors that interfere with your effectiveness and cause conflict, and take on a series of costly and risky, effective behaviors. In short, do the things that will make you more influential in influencing the behaviors of others.

There are two general kinds of appropriate perceptions to put in someone's head that connect what you want with their values. Up until now, I have for the most part used the phrase "serve their values." That can have two quite different, indeed almost opposed, meanings. You can get someone to do something you want by having them perceive that, if they engage in the behavior, they will experience a net increase of value satisfaction in their lives. This is the positive approach, because they have a positive reason for doing what you want. You can also influence others by having people perceive that if they don't engage in the behavior you want, they will experience a net loss of value satisfaction in their lives. This is the negative approach, because people respond to it an effort to avoid losing value satisfaction. Each can be effective. Each approach can be used morally or immorally. There is no moral superiority of positive over negative. The con artist, the cheat, the liar, all use the positive approach.

There is, nonetheless, a pragmatic reason for not using the negative approach, or, more accurately, for not being perceived to be using the negative approach. Each of us learned, early in life, how to cope with the negative approach to human behavior. We have at least three coping mechanisms and each works to the disadvantage of the influencer.

• You try to get out from under the person's influence. If you succeed, the person doesn't influence you. Even if you don't succeed, you are using your energy in a way that is in opposition to the person's values.

• Whenever a person is perceived to be using the negative approach on you, you tend to compute the minimally acceptable behavior you can give them. If you have ever tried to get your children to clean their rooms, you know the technique. You threaten to ground them, to take away their allowance, or the like. They then treat you to a spectacle called "minimum energy in slow motion." It may not be as obvious when other people do it, because they don't want to expose themselves to punishments and reveal their motives, but they are going to give a minimum of the desired behavior and give it grudgingly.

• Finally, you perceive the negative approach as an assault on your self-esteem and sense of autonomy. You are reminded that somebody is ready, able, and willing to take value satisfaction away from you. It doesn't feel good. You are being forced to choose between two undesirable states, two losses of value satisfaction. The loss you think you will sustain if you do what they want and the greater loss you think you will sustain if you don't. In order to reassert your self-esteem, because you don't like to use your time and energy to cut your losses, you may try to get even at some later date. Use of the negative approach runs the risk of making for you an enemy, someone who derives value satisfaction from depriving you of value satisfaction. Enemies have long memories and great creativity. Some people go out of their way to make enemies; they speak with pride of having enemies. I think that is foolish. Life is difficult enough without having people out there ready, willing, and able to take value satisfaction from you if given a relative low-cost and low-risk opportunity to do so.

A true story will illustrate the danger of creating enemies. I was in Chicago's O'Hare Airport a few years ago on my way back to Philadelphia. As I approached the airline counter that served multiple gates, I saw a businessman already there who was absolutely out of control, screaming, cursing, and threatening the woman behind the counter. She handled it beautifully, smiling and never getting rattled. She assured him she understood and would do what she could. She was using what I call "The Managerial Martial Arts." He finally huffed off to his gate. He was going to JFK in New York. I walked up and complimented her on averting a potential conflict. I told her she had used a classic technique as well as I had ever seen it done. She thanked me, but said she had been trained for just such situations. The staff had gone through simulation and role playing to learn how to deal with just such occurrences. She also said that if it really got bad, she had an emergency button to push for assistance. I said that I knew all of that but that I was still impressed—that I was certain many of her colleagues wouldn't have pulled it off as well as she had. Then she smiled, looked to the left and right and said quietly, "Did you notice that the gentleman was on his way to JFK in New York." I said, "yes." She then said, "He doesn't know it yet, but his baggage is on its way to Bangkok."

Always remember—anyone who can engage in behavior to serve your values can, if they wish, engage in behavior that threatens your values. You don't want to give them a reason to do so. On the basis of these problems that are inherent in the use of the negative approach, I am going to provide a model only of the positive approach to human influence.

What follows is an equation for human information processing. It is a model (albeit simplified) of the way in which people evaluate your attempts to influence them. It is a guideline for constructing the data fragments of your behavior to increase the likelihood those fragments will penetrate their filters, touch their values, and elicit the behavior you want. These guidelines flow from all the previous discussions of values and perceptions, power and influence in this book. I do not promise success every time if these guidelines are followed, even if they are followed rigorously. But I do promise that you will increase your effectiveness and that you will activate a potential for success that cannot be achieved in the absence of the guidelines.

Guideline One:
CAPABILITY

Whenever you are trying to influence someone and you think it may be difficult for them or you are meeting resistance or delay, ask yourself this very important question: Can they do what I want them to do? Do they have the capability? That means, do they know what to do; do they have the competence, (the knowledge and the skill, the resources, the time, the energy, the authority), and the self-confidence to do it? If any one of these qualities is lacking, you are not going to get the desired behavior. There are people who are competent but not very self-confident. If you ask someone to do something and they do not have confidence that they can, they don't say that they're incompetent or unskilled or afraid. And they're not going to try to do it, because they believe they can't. That course risks failure for them. So they fudge and play games and engage in all kinds of mechanisms that irritate you. If you put some pressure on them, their behavior becomes even more bizarre. There are also people who are self-confident but not very competent. They will try anything. Fail at what they do and then rationalize their failure. A helpful goal for you is to ensure, however best it can be achieved, that people have the requisite knowledge of the behavior as well as the competence and self-confidence to perform it. If not, provide whatever is missing in them or look for some alternative way to get your values served.

Guideline Two:
PERCEPTION OF POTENTIAL VALUE SATISFACTION

Often, there is no good reason for people to do something that we ask for. They do not perceive any potential value satisfaction in what we are asking them to do. It will not contribute to their security, fun, achievement, or success. What we are asking them to do may also be irritating, inconvenient, costly, or risky. If we want them to do as we want, we will have to attach perceived potential value satisfaction to it. That means for example that you will owe them something if they take it on. You put some chits on the table, and maybe now they have a reason to comply. People do things for other people because they like them, respect them, or owe them. They do things for people whom they want to owe them. They do things in anticipation of success, achievement, recognition, gratitude, fun, excitement, approval, etc. Either you get them to perceive these as potential value satisfactions as consequences of the behavior or you are unlikely to influence them.

You gain power by putting these perceptions of potential value satisfaction in people's heads. If they work with you, they get recognized. They get appreciated. They get approval. You place those perceptions in their heads by the patterns of your behavior over time. You have to convince them, by your behavior, that there is a potential for some such value satisfaction if they engage in the behavior that you want.

Guideline Three:
PERCEPTION OF THE PROBABILITY OF VALUE SATISFACTION
You cannot influence the behavior of others in the absence of perceived trust. People will do things for people they trust that they will do for no one else. Trust is enormously powerful and equally fragile. Like Humpty Dumpty—once broken, it is very difficult to put back together again. Trust is so important in human relationships that we have had to invent a huge, complex, and very expensive mechanism for situations in which people don't trust each other. It's called contract law. The only reason for contract law is to satisfy guideline three, so that strangers, or people who know and don't trust each other, can still engage in transactions. It may not feel good to engage in behaviors that increase the perception of our trustworthiness by those we wish to influence. We don't think we should have to do that. But, if you want power, you have to do it. For example, when you do something you promised to do, write a note telling the person it's taken care of. That person thereby receives a data fragment that reminds them that when you say you'll do something, you do it. You can be trusted. I cannot overestimate how powerful a tool this is in the pursuit of power.

Guideline Four:
PERCEPTION OF COST
When you are trying to influence someone, they will perceive some cost to them of doing it. Time, energy, opportunity. Whatever they could have been doing to gain value satisfaction instead of what you want them to do. Their perception of cost may be greatly exaggerated (and often is). But, you must deal with it as it is in their perceptions, not in your sense of what is realistic or reasonable. We can usually reduce their perception of risk by taking some or all of it on ourselves. But we don't want to do that. We don't think we should have to. So we tend to do what is low cost and easy and curse them when they don't do what we want. When attempting to lower people's perceptions of cost, try to think of ways to give them options and a sense of control over what you want them to do. The more sense of options and control they perceive they have, the lower they will weight their perceived costs.

Influencing Them To Do What You Want Them To Do

Guideline Five:
PERCEPTION OF RISK
The only difference between cost and risk is the perceived probability of the loss of value satisfaction. If someone perceives a loss to be 100 percent probable, they count it as a cost. If the perceived probability is any less than that, they perceive it as a risk. The person you seek to influence is very likely to perceive some risk, some potential loss of value satisfaction, in doing what you want. Maybe they think they are getting in over their heads. Maybe they think they are writing a blank check. Maybe they think they will be censored by their associates. Maybe they are concerned that if they do it this time, they will always be the one to be called on to make the sacrifice, to take on the distasteful task. Perception of risk is often difficult to deal with, because it is usually hidden from the influencer and may even be nothing more than a fuzzy sense of "this doesn't feel right to me" in the influencee. It is often exaggerated even more than a sense of cost. But, it must be dealt with if you are to succeed in influence. Try to take some of the risk onto yourself. Try to spread it across several people, so that the person you are trying to influence feels more comfortable with what you want. Interestingly, you can often get two or three people do something no one of them is willing to do alone simply because they feel lower risk in the company of others.

CONCLUSION
That's my equation, my model, for human information processing. That's how I think everybody processes, usually subconsciously, whenever anybody tries to influence them. No matter how subconscious the process is, we go through those five conditions and they are the ones you must attend to if you are to increase your interpersonal and group effectiveness. There is a difficulty, of course. Those trying to influence others and those being influenced are operating in exactly opposite directions. When we are influencers, we tend to exaggerate guidelines two and three and discount guidelines four and five. The influencee discounts two and three (based on past experience) while exaggerating four and five. That is the explanation for the frequency with which we find people unreasonable when we are trying to influence their behavior. There are hundreds, perhaps even thousands, of behaviors you can engage in, in a given situation, to alter each of those perceptions in people's heads, but they all have costs and risks attached to them for you. None of them will work 100 percent of the time, but they do work more powerfully than whatever you are doing now. You have to assess the costs and risks to you, but, in the end, you have to accept them if you are interested in influencing other people and thereby gaining power in the service of your values.

A FINAL SUMMARY

Behavior is a function of people's capability plus their perception of potential value satisfaction, multiplied by their perception of the probability of gaining the value satisfaction if they engage in the behavior minus their perception of the costs and perception of the risks they will have to bear by engaging in the behavior. Behavior = Capability + (Perception of Potential Value Satisfaction x Perception of the Probability of Value Satisfaction) — (Perception of Cost and Perception of Risk). Influence (and power) are nothing more or less than your ability to affect those five states, four of which are perceptions—personal, fragile, subjective, idiosyncratic, arbitrary, and infinitely malleable states in the other's head. All that you have available to you to affect those perceptions are the data fragments of your own behavior. If carefully crafted, they are more than adequate. Your power is limited only by your willingness to accept the personal costs and risks inherent in effective behaviors.

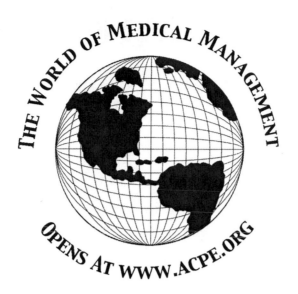

THE WORLD OF MEDICAL MANAGEMENT OPENS AT WWW.ACPE.ORG

If you're already in medical management or are in the process of pursuing a medical management career, information on the tools for success are at http://www/acpe/org.

The ACPE Publications Catalog.

Peruse descriptions of the many medical management offerings of the College and order copies on line.

Line-Up of Educational Offerings.

Complete descriptions and advanced schedules for the College's nationally recognized medical management curriculum are provided. Also described are College-sponsored advanced degree programs.

Myriad Ways to Manage and Advance Your Career.

Up-to-the-minute position postings, services for resume construction, and other career services are designed to promote medical management and help physicians move into management positions.

This is a jam-packed Web site.
See for yourself.
http://www.acpe.org

We've Made Your Mouse Mighty!

Now, at the click of a mouse, you can gain access to the latest thinking on critical issues in medical management. All of it comes to you in *Click*, the American College of Physician Executives' on-line journal for physician executives. You can access *Click* at www.acpe.org/click.

- In-depth articles that explore the leading edge of medical management issues and trends.

- Feedback mechanism for comments on an article or on your efforts in the area covered by an article.

- Additional resources on the topic covered by an article.

- Access to comments from reviewers and readers of the article.

Don't take our word for it. The best way to experience this new publishing venture is to see it first-hand. Take your mouse on a visit to *Click*.

Printed in the United States
128838LV00002B/67-93/A

9 780924 674129